Fitness Frauds
Exposing the Truth About Drugs, Lies, and Flex Appeal

Bobby Whisnand

Inspire On Purpose Publishing
Irving, Texas

Fitness Frauds: Exposing the Truth About Drugs, Lies, and Flex Appeal

Inspire on Purpose Publishing
Irving, Texas
(888) 403-2727
https://inspireonpurpose.com
The Platform Publisher™
"Changing Lives With Words"

Printed in the United States of America

Library of Congress Control Number: 2017958215
Softcover ISBN-13: 978-1-941782-44-6

Also by Bobby Whisnand

It's All Heart

A Body To Die For: The Painful Truth About Exercise

12 Rounds: A Day to Day Guide to a Better Life

Contents

Introduction

Fitness: A multi-billion-dollar industry built on the hopes and dreams of millions of people who want to look good and live longer.

From the occasional exerciser, to the hard-core, seven-days-a-week gym rat, to the folks who are allergic to exercise, people all over the world are spending billions of dollars a year to jump head first into the fountain of fit. And waiting in every gym to sell you a six-pack are personal trainers, exercise class instructors, and "overnight health coaches" promising to add time and quality to your life as they take you to the land of lean and ripped.

What about bodybuilders, fitness pageant contestants, extremely fit looking individuals, and the sixty-year-olds with twenty-year-old bodies we see all over social media, on TV, and in the gym? With the bodies they have, one would be crazy not to take their fitness advice, especially because they're all natural, right?

If that's not enough, there are hundreds of thousands of fitness companies and individuals advertising simple yet miraculous exercise equipment, the latest and greatest one-size-fits-all exercise programs (before and after pics included), and magic fitness pills. And if you order "right now" (insert siren), you can have guaranteed success just like the other people who have used these products, all in a matter of weeks!

Or if you want to put your wellness hopes in a bottle of pills or a bucket of powder, you can trudge your way through the self-help supplement industry and hope you find health instead of a holistic hoax. If unhealthy eating is your biggest challenge, not to worry; we have an entire food industry offering up "healthy alternatives and solutions" in grocery stores and restaurants all over the world. And if accountability, calorie counting, and celebrity-endorsed weight-loss plans are your choice for wellness, there are countless programs ready to help you fit back into your high school jeans in no time. With all of this help, instruction, and can't-miss fitness methods available, we should all have no problem being lean, muscular, fit, and ready to hit the beach, right?

This is exactly what the fitness industry wants you to believe—that if you exercise and eat like those in the industry tell you to, beast mode will be your new happy place, and you will end up looking all fit and ripped up, just like your trainer does. And this, my friend, is the biggest scam going on in our world today, and millions are falling for it.

First of all, most "certified" personal trainers, exercise class instructors, and boot camp coaches have a greater knack for ripping rotators, breaking backs, and killing cartilage than building healthy bodies. But hey, you really killed that workout.

Second, before you emulate the exercise routines and diets of competitive bodybuilders, women's figure and swimsuit contestants, or the big, strong, and completely unnatural looking people walking around the gym, just know the "juice" doesn't fall far from the tree. There's a lot more going on with them than exercise and eating right.

In addition, TV, magazines, and the always credible world of social media will attempt to lure you every few seconds with amazingly fraudulent fitness transformation stories, and, of course, those "one-of-a-kind" products and methods that work miracles.

And the wild world of supplements—between almost nonexistent regulations and ingredient roulette, what you think you're putting into your body and what's really going in there are two vastly different things. Don't forget about the food industry: Making you healthy isn't the top priority; making money is. From low-fat claims to visions of chickens running free, food companies use labels of lies to hide unhealthy truths about the foods they're putting on the shelves, as they attempt to remove your doubts while emptying your wallets.

And last, the big business of weight loss is causing a lot of people to lose a lot more than weight, although spokespeople with emotional testimonials will try to convince you otherwise. Or you could forget all of this and just listen to the millions of differing opinions on whether to eat like a caveman, graze like a cow, or something bizarre in between.

The fact is, the very industry that is supposed to lead us to true, safe, and productive ways to better our health is instead lying through its biceps and feeding us a bunch of bull.

I've been in the fitness industry since 1990, and I've witnessed hundreds of trainers and class instructors turn thousands of healthy bodies into walking orthopedic nightmares, all because of an incredibly high level of incompetence in functional and safe exercise. Those little tweaks of pain, that swelling in your joints, and that stiffness in your lower back? All normal, right? Just push through the pain, bro.

And then there are the drugs. From the early '90s to the early 2000s, I personally witnessed the rise and fall of one of the biggest steroid rings ever, leading to prison for some and death for others. I've watched hundreds of men and women over the years make amazing transformations in a matter of weeks and listened as they told everyone that all they do is work out and eat right. The funny thing is, amid all their denial of using drugs, I personally witnessed them taking secret deliveries of their "supplements" because most of these exchanges occurred right there on the gym floor. Although a much wider scope of people across the fitness industry today are taking drugs, it's a lot more discrete, but the proof is glaring from one end to the next.

I've also watched the fitness industry get really good over the last twenty years at pumping up user success stories in advertising campaigns. You know what I'm talking about: the before and after pics, the "I've tried everything in the world, and this is the only thing that works" testimonials, and, of course, the celebrity endorsements.

And then there's the food industry, teaching us how to camouflage bad food with good label tricks—lose twenty pounds in two days—and how to expect that what's good today will be bad tomorrow.

MOST of the fitness industry is built on lies. You can call it stealing, robbing, or cheating—all of which are true— but I'm going to call it what it really is: FRAUD.

Fraud: A false representation of a matter of fact—whether by words or by conduct, by false or misleading allegations, or by concealment of what should have been disclosed—that deceives and is intended to deceive another so that the individual will act upon it to her or his legal injury (as defined by thefreedictionary.com).

Yes, fraud is a strong word, but we are talking about the fitness industry, so a "strong" word is necessary. The fitness industry is out of shape—loafing, as my dad would say—and once I pull back the curtains to expose its many empty promises and pharmaceutical fakeness, you'll see its true colors, and a lot of things will definitely start to make sense. My goals with this book are simple: to expose the personal training and exercise instructor industry for what it really is; to uncover the truth about drug use in all areas of fitness; to show you what's hiding behind the smoke, mirrors, and masquerades within fitness advertisements; to clean up the dirty truth behind the food, nutrition, and weight-loss industries; and to give you my solutions to right the ship of fitness and wellness altogether.

There's one thing I want you to know before you go any further: Exercising how you want or taking drugs to help things along is absolutely your right and your business; that's not my point with this book. But when fraudulent means and methods are used to make personal gains at the expense of others, especially when it comes to health, the crooks need to be exposed.

In my first chapter, I throw a forceful punch at the very industry of which I have been a part since 1990: personal training and exercise instructors. Actually, we should change the title "personal trainer" to "personal injurer," and once you read through this chapter, you'll see exactly why. I'm going to explain in great detail why many trainers and other exercise instructors should be given stock in joint replacement surgeries because they send an endless supply of patients to orthopedic doctors everywhere. And make sure you listen when a trainer tells you that pain is weakness leaving the body because, while you may not know this, most trainers are almost doctors who can diagnose and treat your injuries. No need to go to the doctor; they can tell you exactly what's wrong, and even better, they can put you through physical therapy (PT) because they've had a lot of experience with the same injury you have. Wow! What a coincidence! And those letters by their name on their business cards showing the different certifications they have? Priceless! And by priceless I mean without value.

In Chapter 2, I will show you just how easy it is to get a personal training or instructor certification and, more importantly, just how insignificant those credentials really are. I'm going to show you exactly what certifications do and do not teach and the really important things most of them miss. Certifications could be the right start when beginning a career in personal training or exercise class instruction, but most of them are nothing but certified poppycock. Personal training and exercise instructors aren't the only ones beating up bodies, busting ligaments, and giving false hope; there's a huge glorified part of the fitness industry full of fake flex appeal taking center stage that has its hands dirty as well.

The appeal of the amazing physiques we see in bodybuilding/fitness pageants, on TV, in movies, all over social media, and walking around in the local gym is completely understandable. But what the general public mostly misunderstands is that exercise and eating right aren't the only things these folks did to get those bodies. I'm talking about the almost 100 percent likelihood that anabolic steroids and other drugs were involved in their "diet and exercise" routines. In Chapter 3, I'm going to show you just how prevalent drugs are within the fitness industry, both in and out of physique competitions, and how this is falsely shaping and dictating what being fit should really look like.

> From the professional athlete to the sixty-year-old women's tennis player at the country club, the cocktails are flowing, but the juice they're drinking isn't from any blender.

Everyone wants to find the fountain of youth, and from the looks of things, they've found something all right, but it's not youth that's flowing through it. I highly doubt the fitness industry is full of chemistry majors, but the lab is open 24/7 and it's doing very well.

Steroids and other illegal "fitness" drugs are flowing through the fitness industry like pre-workout and protein drinks.

In Chapter 4, I'm going to show you the exact drugs being taken by countless people across the fitness industry, the different groups of "fitness enthusiasts" who are taking them, exactly what these drugs do, and where they come from. Now, how do we get all of these people to admit they're taking drugs to get their fake fit look? Do we just hand them each a little cup and say, "Fill 'er up"?

The odds of someone admitting to using drugs to enhance their look is almost zero. They simply don't want people to know that their athletic prowess, their three-month amazing physical transformation, or that newly found thirty pounds of lean muscle is fake. So how do we know who's on drugs and who's not? In Chapter 5,

I'm going to show you how drug testing is spotty at best, and at the same time, the means and methods many people use to fake a drug test—you won't believe some of them! Lying about drug use is commonplace in the fitness industry, but what about fitness advertisements? Are the ads lying too?

Chapter 6 takes on another huge chunk of the fitness industry that's faking it: fitness advertisements. We've all seen the wonder workouts and miracle machine commercials and heard the screams and sirens about can't-miss successes and money-back guarantees. So are these lies too, or is what we're seeing for real? What do you think? In this chapter, I'm going to show you how fitness advertisements use smoke, mirrors, and masquerades to pull fast ones and get you to buy into these worthless products and promises. Speaking of cheap, worthless, and shady, how many supplements are in your kitchen cabinet or gym bag right now?

Supplements are a multi-billion-dollar business that continues to stock shelves with powders, pills, and snake oils, all designed to make everything about you better. From proprietary blends to multi-vitamin mega-mixtures, everything you'll ever need to take your fitness and health to the next fifteen levels is available on just about every corner, even in grocery stores. If only we had a supplement lie detector to scan each supplement. Do you think it would go off much? In Chapter 7, I'm going to give you my "warning label" to look for when buying supplements because, just like the fitness industry itself, very few are really effective, some we just don't know, and most aren't worth a dime. To top off this chapter, I'm going to show you how the world of multi-level marketing has its hand in the dubious distribution of supplements and why you should be leery of their stories and products. Most supplements aren't what they say, but there's yet another industry feeding us a load.

In a grocery store near you, the food industry is stocking its fakeness up and down every aisle, hoping you'll trust their labels and ignore the fine details. The "fake and bake" food business is thriving because millions are falling for labels of lies and camouflaged ingredients.

> Whether it's the sweet stuff, the fat stuff, or the "all-natural" stuff, food companies do a great job of hiding the truth about their products and are hoping the only thing you're contemplating is paper or plastic.

In Chapter 8, you're going to get a very detailed look into exactly how food companies mislead and fake us out with their clever labels and packaging, and more importantly, how to win at the "whole" food fight. Speaking of a food fight, there are plenty of big business weight-loss companies promising to stand side-by-side with you in your fight to lose weight. Can they really help you win, or are they just good at helping you lose all the way around?

When it comes to pulling a fast one, weight-loss programs, miracle diets, and the always open "social media nutrition store" all tie for the blue ribbon. Oh, there are plenty of ways to lose weight, but chances are, weight isn't the only thing you're going to lose. The "ten pounds in two days," the "no exercise required," and the "carbs are bad" diets are all jockeying for the lead in the "we're full of it race." In Chapter 9, I'm going to show you where many diet programs go wrong and how to determine if a weight-loss company is good at losing in all the right places. Cleaning your plate is a tough job under any circumstances, but when you add all the other fraudulent acts running rampant across our fitness and wellness industry, the job becomes something much greater and enduring.

It's a shame that this book even has to be written. Here I am taking an industry, which is supposed to be built on helping people live longer and better lives, and I'm knocking the legs out from under it. Yes, that's exactly what I'm doing. Someone needs to stand up, call out the liars, and expose an upside-down, wasting industry for what it really is. I've been on the front lines of the fitness industry for nearly three decades, and I can say with 100-percent certainty that most of what I have seen over these years is anything but healthy, and for the most part, it's fraudulent. On the outside, the fitness industry looks like a big bundle of happy health, encouraging everyone to come join the fun. But on the inside, it's a broken and twisted mess, hoping you never see the truth.

> *"The fitness industry is a lot like politics. They both start out with a lot of hot air and promises, only to end up as a big fat lie."*
>
> *~ Bobby Whisnand*

1 Fit-Less Instructors
Killer Workouts or Killing Joints?

Personal trainers, group exercise instructors, boot camp generals, and "overnight fitness coaches" all over the world are pumped and ready to push you through the pain, baby! But it will cost you. I'm not talking about gym memberships or your ten-pack of personal training sessions. I'm talking about the price you're most likely to pay for bulging discs, jacked-up joints, and a future full of medical bills, all because your trainer convinced you to push through those sharp pains in your lower back and those little aches and pains in your knees and shoulders that make you walk funny and unable to wash your own hair. But it's cool, man, and definitely worth the pain because your instructor says you're killing it! The question is, what exactly are you killing?

This first chapter is the hard-hitting truth about the fraudulent and outrageously unhealthy acts of personal trainers, exercise class instructors, and other pretend fitness experts, and exactly how they rob you of a lot more than money. First, I'm going to show you how most trainers and instructors don't know half of what they pretend to know about exercise and nutrition, and how they conceal their ignorance from their paying clients. Second, I'm going to uncover the costliest mistakes made by most fitness instructors (you'd better update your health insurance). And if that isn't enough, I'm going to expose how trainers and instructors play doctor by not only diagnosing an injury (one they more than likely caused) but also by actually prescribing treatment as well. Sounds like a double dip to me. And to top all of this off, I'm going to tell you a few horror stories of personal trainer mishaps that ended very badly for the clients. Let's just say the clients didn't walk out of the gym on their own; the paramedics rolled them out.

I've been in the personal trainer industry since the caveman era. I've watched hundreds of different trainers and instructors pound the life out of their clients' bodies and receive praise for making them practically have to crawl out of the gym after their workouts. I've seen crazy and ridiculous made-up exercises that would make the circus come recruiting; I've witnessed (and unfortunately heard) countless torn muscles and ruptured ligaments pop from "one more rep"; and I've seen thousands of backs broken from horrible squatting and deadlifting form, all at the hands of personal trainers and exercise instructors. But don't trainers and instructors know how to perform exercises correctly? I mean, they're certified and they're in great shape, right? We will get into that in the next chapter, but as far as knowing how to perform exercises correctly, they either don't have a clue, or they just don't care.

So how much do trainers and instructors really know about exercise, physiology, and nutrition? A lot less than they lead you to believe. There are a few trainers out there who are very knowledgeable about the human body and exercise, but most instructors aren't. And even if they do have a good handle on physiology and proper exercise, the chances of them applying it to their training methods are slim to none. So how do they hide their ignorance? Easy. They lie and make stuff up. Nice, huh? Even though most trainers and exercise instructors are certified, they are ignorant on the workings of the human body. As you will see in the next chapter, certifications don't mean much at all, and as far as knowing the body, the trainer will have to use a coloring book to show you.

When you read a trainer's personal bio, you'll see the impressive letters signifying their certifications and their countless years of exercise experience, but what you won't see is a list of injuries they've caused. They'll throw around a few key muscle names like biceps femoris and vastus medialis, and a few terms like sagittal plane and pronation, but for the most part, they're clueless. They may know a few other muscles, but it's mostly just chest, shoulders, triceps, legs, back, biceps, and abs. They know where the machines are on the gym floor, can count reps, and will tell you when you're out of sessions. I will say that trainers and instructors are great sources of accountability for their clients, but the crazy thing is, instructors are the ones who need to be held accountable the most. So do you want to have some fun, flip the script, and watch trainers and class instructors sweat for a change? Ask them my Fit 4 Fail questions, but don't hold your breath; it may take them a while to respond.

Fit 4 Fail – Four questions every trainer or instructor should be able to answer correctly

Question 1. Can you explain which muscles I'm working with this exercise?

Don't let them slide with just saying legs, chest, abdominals, etc. The body has 640 muscles, and although most of them are very hard to remember, your trainer should at least be able to tell you the main ones along with the muscles that make up a group, like quadriceps, triceps, and (for certain) the rotator cuff. Yes, definitely ask them to tell you the four muscles of the rotator cuff. I wouldn't expect much here. They may even say rotator "cup" instead of cuff, which is a dead giveaway of their lack of knowledge. While you're at it, ask them to explain antagonist muscles and how they work together. Maybe you could give them a chart of all the muscles for Christmas. Ego check in three... two... one.

Question 2. Why are we doing this particular exercise, and how does it benefit me?

Now we're really going to get somewhere. They won't have their cheat sheet for this one either, so be prepared for answers like, "It's a good exercise; everybody does it," "I do the same exercise and it works for me," "It makes you really sore," and "It uses your core a lot." Don't settle for these garbage answers. Make them explain in rational detail, or watch them stand there and look stupid. While you're at it, get them to explain what constitutes the body's "core." If you really want to stir the pot, do the research yourself on a particular exercise and when they can't answer, answer it for them. You may hurt their ego, but that's better than them hurting you.

Question 3. How sore should I be getting, and is it OK to work out sore muscles?

Oh yes, the glorified BS of extreme soreness. Making you walk like a zombie for three days and causing you to take pain relievers and anti-inflammatories because of intense soreness is not a great idea. But somehow this extreme soreness is looked upon as an indicator of a great workout.

In the land of personal injury—I mean personal training—making clients so sore that they can't walk right, sit on the commode, or lift a coffee cup seems to be the goal.

Maybe these instructors are certified soreness experts, and certification makes it totally acceptable, right? Seriously, extreme soreness is looked upon like a badge of honor for both the client and the trainer, and it's absolutely ridiculous. Should you be this sore? No way. Never.

Here's another great question for you to ask: Why is it good for me to be this sore? The answer you'll probably get is, "It means we worked your entire muscle really good and broke down the muscle really good too." Broke is the key word here. What about working out a sore muscle? I can tell you the answer you'll get from that question too: "We're going to work the soreness out. You need to get the lactic acid out of your muscle." And yet another lie born from ignorance. Look, any soreness that lasts for more than seventy-two hours and/or causes you to modify the way you move during everyday activities is way too much. Light to moderate soreness for forty-eight hours is perfect. Call them out on this!

Question 4. Is joint pain normal during and after exercise, especially as I get older?

Your trainer or instructor should know that any amount of pain is not good, but most are strong proponents of what I call the Beast Mode Prophecy. This question is easy for them to answer with the age-old saying, "No pain, no gain," or the popular slogan, "Pain is weakness leaving the body." I wish I could take a bullhorn into the gym so that every time I hear it said I could yell, "Liar!" I guess if you look at the way most trainers and class instructors treat their clients' bodies during their sessions then joint pain should be expected. Here we have another great question for you to ask: Explain to me why my joint pain is healthy? Be prepared for the pause, blank stare, and then the ever so intelligent answer, "It means your muscles are tired or you have an old injury." As far as pain being a part of getting older, this is a lame, BS excuse that gets way too much credit. Even if you have a pre-existing injury, there are ways to modify your exercises so you have no pain. Plain and simple, you shouldn't hurt during or after exercise. If you do, it's your fault now.

There are hundreds of other questions you could ask, but there's really no point; you'll get the same vague, pointless, and wrong answers to them too. Lying and making up pseudo-answers are two things trainers and instructors should definitely add to their bios, but there's more—a whole lot more. And guess what? I've got them all ready for you to see right now. Let's take a closer look at exactly what trainers and exercise instructors are doing during their "go hard or go home" sessions.

Why do you think exercise equipment breaks? It's not because it's used a lot. It's because the equipment gets abused, pounded, jerked, and slammed, just like the bodies using it. It's one thing to see someone exercising incorrectly by themselves, but it's a whole bigger issue when there's a trainer or instructor standing right beside them and not correcting anything. But I see it all day every day and have since I entered this business in 1990. And if you take a look in a gym, inside an exercise class, or do a slow drive by a boot camp, you'll see why joint replacements are sky rocketing and why pain medication is as common as vitamins.

And right there like a drill sergeant is a trainer or instructor killing cartilage with every rep.

You may not believe it's this bad, and I'd like to be able to tell you it isn't, but it is. OK, I've waited long enough. It's time for my first story, and it's a good one. I was warming up on a bike at the gym and right beside me was a trainer talking to his client, and this is the conversation that ensued:

> *Trainer: Hey, you ready to roll?*

> *Client: Not really. My knee is swollen and hurts from what we did yesterday.*

> *Trainer: No way; we didn't do anything to hurt your knee. It must have been something you did after your workout.*

> *Client: No, it was during the workout when I was squatting. I even told you it felt weird and hurt after our last set.*

> *Trainer: I don't remember that but we will fix it.*

> *Client: How are we going to fix it? Shouldn't we leave it alone for a while?*

Trainer: No way; that's the worst thing we could do. We need to get it moving or it will stiffen up. Let's do what we did yesterday except with lighter weights, and then we'll stretch it out. You'll be fine, and it will feel better tomorrow. Don't worry; I deal with this all the time.

It took everything I had not to call that trainer an idiot and walk the client out of the gym. I watched them closely to see what was going to happen, and guess what exercise they did first? Squats! And after only two grueling repetitions, the client dropped the bar, limped to a bench, sat down, and held her knee in pain. They applied ice, and a few gym employees graciously helped her to her car. I never saw her after that day. I hope she was OK, but I doubt it.

Now might be a good time to pause and explain why I don't intervene when I witness these injuries-in-the-making. In a nutshell, because calling out a trainer would, unfortunately, be counterproductive and ineffective on several levels. First, I would be alienated at my place of work, to put it bluntly. This is the place where I spend ten or twelve hours a day, and you can imagine the payback that would most certainly ensue. Second, my attempts to correct other trainers would most likely be ignored anyway, since EVERYONE is using the same injury-causing form and technique, and it's all viewed as normal, just like pain. Last, the relationship between a trainer and client is somewhat intimate. The client is invested, emotionally and physically, which creates a bond that's almost impossible to break. Writing this book was my way of educating the public about what's wrong and what's right in the world of fitness so clients (and potential clients) can call out incompetent trainers themselves.

Believe me, I see idiotic behavior from trainers every day. So what exactly are trainers and class instructors doing that is so bad? Just about everything, but I'll give you only the ones I see the most in my Methods to the Madness section.

Methods to the Madness

Take a look at these popular training methods most often used by trainers and instructors, but watch out for flying cartilage and busted ligaments!

Turbo Lifting – I think trainers have an undisclosed contest to see whose client can get through a set of fifteen reps the fastest. If you aren't taking four to five seconds and pausing at the top and bottom of each repetition, you're going too fast. I never see trainers telling anyone to slow down. All I hear is, "Yeah, beast mode!" and "You killed it!" And then the client is so worn out that they slam the machine or free weights down. I don't know if I should feel sorrier for the client or the weights. Speed racing through reps will only lead to one thing: an orthopedic surgeon's office.

The Swing and Jerk – You know what I mean. The trainer lets the client use their entire body to swing or jerk the weight up just to say they did it. This usually happens with bicep curls, shoulder presses, and side lateral raises. Oh man, I've seen people almost bend in half just to get the weight up or finish that last rep. And the trainer is full of encouragement and praise for them lifting a heavier weight. And the L-5 disc will bulge in three... two... one. Welcome to the wonderful world of sciatica! Is your trainer paying for your surgery?

The Camel – Also known as the rounded back. This one occurs mostly when a client is squatting or deadlifting (especially straight-leg deadlifting), and from start to finish, their back is humped like a camel. And yet again, the trainer is yelling for them to get it up as they "spot" them through a disastrous lift. But it's OK; that sciatic nerve pain is only down one leg for now, and the client has thirty-two—make that thirty-one—more discs that aren't ruptured, yet!

The Knee Ripper – This is the most popular technique being taught today. You can see this particular method being used mostly on the leg extension machine, or during lunges or squats in most exercise classes and most certainly in your local boot camp. When doing the leg extension, trainers often have clients combine the turbo lift and the swing and jerk, just to make certain that the cartilage in the knees gets a thorough pounding. If you want to see the knee ripper combined with the camel, hang out by the squat racks, or watch trainers and their clients when they do lunges.

Knees way out over the toes, the tendon-busting bounce at the bottom, and the hump from hell curving their backs are all prime examples of proper form on display by a certified personal trainer or group exercise instructor.

This gives getting ripped a whole new meaning. Hey, did you know the circus is in town? It's always in town.

Circus Auditions

Oh yes, let the entertainment begin! Circus acts should take place under a big top, not under a barbell. I have to admit, although the clown acts I see from trainers and instructors are going to most likely hurt their clients, it's quite entertaining to see some of the exercises the trainers make up.

I keep waiting for the circus music to start, the little car to roll in, and all the clowns to spill out when I see the twisted ball of wrong that trainers have their clients do.

And you can see the look of dismay on a client's face when the trainer shows them the "act" they want performed. Look, improving body balance should be a part of everyone's fitness plan, but when the risk of an exercise outweighs the reward, it becomes stupid, plain and simple. And by stupid, I mean completely without intelligence. Here are a few examples of the circus acts I've seen trainers make their clients perform; the only things missing are the funny music and the big red noses.

The Balancing DUMBbell Act

Standing on dumbbells doing squats, deadlifts, or any other exercises is a horrible and completely idiotic idea, as is doing push-ups on dumbbells so the shoulders can really take a ripping. Yep, stupid and completely without sense. Just the other day I was watching what was supposed to be a fitness evaluation with a trainer and client, and when I saw what they were doing, I knew it was not going to end well. The trainer had the client stand on top of dumbbells to perform a squat. First of all, the dumbbells were the little bitty ones, like two-pounders, and they were rolling back and forth under her feet as she was valiantly trying to balance. And then she attempted to do a body weight squat. Although it was very shaky, she made the first squat, but on the next one, the dumbbell under her right foot slipped, out went her right leg, and down she went. That was it; she limped out and was done. I've also seen push-ups on dumbbells go wrong, injuring shoulders. But it was all supervised by a personal trainer, so it was just an unavoidable accident, right? I don't usually reference other fitness sources for various reasons but considering the topic of performing exercises on an unstable surface, I have one that is perfectly relevant. In a *Men's Fitness* article, "The Stupid Things Bad Trainers Say," the editors listed, "Squat on an unstable surface for more core work."[1] The article went on to mention a couple of studies that debunk the notion that squatting on an unstable surface is beneficial. Good work, *Men's Fitness!*

The Flop-A-Thon

This is where the client gets in a pull-up position and kicks, flops, and jerks their way to a pull-up. Yes, it looks as bad as it sounds and completely wreaks havoc on the shoulder joints. But the trainer says everyone is doing it (including themselves), and it's completely safe, so it must be good. Almost everyone else who's watching this sad excuse for a pull-up is thinking the same thing I am, "What the hell are they doing?"

The Lumbar Leveler

Also known as the reverse hack squat. This is where you get into the hack squat machine facing inward instead of facing outward like normal, and squat away. Sometimes I think I can hear the clients' discs screaming from the rainbow arch in their backs. Why stop at bulging one or two discs? This exercise will get them all. I'd love to have a spine surgeon work out with me, and when we see the lumbar leveler in action, the surgeon could walk over and hand the person a card.

The Cable Carnival

This is where trainers have clients stand on unbalanced platforms like stability or medicine balls, grab cables without handles, and start slinging. That's really the best way I can describe it. It's like a yo-yo going in several different directions at once. But hey, everyone is looking at you and they're impressed. No, they're waiting for something in your body to break. This looks stupid because it is; there are much better, more productive, and safer ways to exercise.

I could go on and on, but I think you get the point. If you missed the last circus when it was in town, not to worry; you can see one every day in your local gym or boot camp. If you're still not sure where to find it, just ask a friendly personal trainer; they'll make sure you get front row seats. What about nutrition advice? Are trainers fouling this up too?

Nutty Nutrition

Man, have I overheard some whoppers when it comes to nutrition advice! This is a very big problem within the fitness instructor business. Trainers are giving completely ridiculous and wrong nutritional advice to clients, and it's absolutely nuts. Why is this happening? Because they simply don't understand nutrition. So exactly where are they going wrong with their "expert" diet advice? Most of the bad advice is centered on carbohydrates. This is the most misunderstood topic in all of nutrition, and if you don't fully understand carbohydrates and how they work in the body, it's best to keep your mouth shut and learn before you mislead others. In Chapter 8, I'm going to uncover the many lies and deceptions within the nutrition and food industry, but for now I'm going to give you a story about a conversation I overheard between a trainer and his client about carbohydrates.

> *Client: I'm still not losing weight after three weeks, and I'm following the diet you gave me 100 percent.*
>
> *Trainer: Are you sure you're following the diet 100 percent?*
>
> *Client: Yes, and I'm hungry all the time. Are you sure I'm eating enough? I feel like my energy has dropped too.*
>
> *Trainer: It just takes time for your body to get used to it. You're probably holding onto water. Yeah, that's it; you're holding water and you're gaining muscle, don't forget that.*
>
> *Client: I just feel like I need to change something. Is there anything else I can change?*
>
> *Trainer: I'll tell you what you can do. Let's go ahead and remove the brown rice from your diet and replace it with sour cream.*
>
> *Client: What? Are you sure? What will that do?*
>
> *Trainer: You'll feel full from the sour cream, and your body will burn more fat without the rice.*
>
> *Client: I don't know, man; that sounds rather extreme. Sour cream? Really?*
>
> *Trainer: Trust me; it'll work.*

This conversation happened. When I heard him tell his client to cut the rice and replace it with sour cream, I was amazed, but not shocked. This is my point: If you don't fully understand carbohydrates, stop talking and start learning. Another area where fitness instructors go terribly awry with their nutrition advice is restricting caloric intake too much. If you were to ask any of my clients about their diets, they'll quickly tell you, "He makes me eat." It's clean eating with meals specifically timed, but you definitely don't go hungry. Diets are tricky, and different individuals require different types of foods in different amounts, but carbohydrates are the key to any diet because they are the quickest and most efficient source of energy for our bodies. Be very leery about nutrition advice, even if it comes from your certified nutritionist trainer. Giving inaccurate nutrition advice is bad enough, but there is something else most trainers are pushing that's even worse.

Personal Pain Pushers

That's it! That's a great new name: Personal Pain Pushers. In fact, the letters PPP should be on nearly every trainer's business card. It's pretty darn accurate from what I can see. I've heard countless clients tell their trainers they are hurt, and what does the trainer say? "Keep going; you'll be fine."

> From muscle strains and tendonitis, to torn ligaments and smashed cartilage, to broken backs and torn biceps, exercise instructors are turning a blind eye to pain while they check their phones for new texts.

But it's nothing that a little ice, an anti-inflammatory, and a knee brace won't fix. Have you ever noticed how many people in the gym wear braces these days? Oh well, that just means they're killing it! From top to bottom and from head to toe, fitness instructors ignore their clients' pain just like they ignore proper exercise techniques. Maybe I missed out on the certified pain management section of my certifications or I learned incorrectly from my physical therapy internships. No, I'm certain. Pain is bad, and if an injury has occurred while you're using a trainer or taking part in an exercise class, it's time to cancel your remaining sessions and save your body and your joints while you can.

Even when a client is so injured that they cannot possibly keep up with their training regimen, the instructor jumps in to save the day. Wouldn't you know it, most fitness instructors are one-stop shops that can not only cause an injury, but also doctor you right up by diagnosing your injury on the spot and prescribing treatment. Lord knows they do have a lot of experience in the injury area.

Playing Doctor

You've seen them on TV with their white coats and stethoscopes, playing the doctor role to a T. They use medical lingo as they walk around administering fake medicine to those who have fallen ill, always throwing out big words to describe injuries and illnesses, and, of course, they're Johnny-on-the-spot with quick diagnoses and treatment plans. The good news is, this is TV, and it's OK to act and portray something you're not. The bad news is there are fitness instructors doing the very same things in gyms, exercise classes, and boot camps all over the world where people's health is truly at stake. Oh, it's going on, and I'm just waiting for the lawsuits to come crashing down, but they never do. You may not know this, but the gym is full of "doctors" wearing workout clothes and stopwatches instead of white coats and stethoscopes. Let's take a deeper look into how trainers are playing doctors, and don't bother checking; they're definitely not on your PPO.

Double Dipping

As bad and scary as this may sound, it's the reality in our fitness instructor world. Not only are fitness instructors causing a lot of injuries by the way they train their clients, but also they are attempting to diagnose and treat their clients. I've witnessed hundreds of clients telling their trainers that they have an injury, and the trainer says the same thing every single time: "Oh, I know what that is. Let me take a look." And the vicious cycle rolls on. First of all, anyone other than a doctor has no business diagnosing anything. And as far as treatment, physical therapists have that locked up. So instead of doing what's right and sending their clients to the doctor to find out exactly what the injury is, the trainers put on their imaginary white coats, put their clients on a massage table, and start poking, bending, and stretching to complete their great act. Are you ready for another crazy story? OK, you asked for it.

A guy I see almost on a daily basis injured his knee by doing one of those balancing circus acts I mentioned previously, and yes, he has a trainer. He came back several times after his injury per his trainer's advice and wouldn't you know it, the knee got worse—much worse. Wow! How could that have possibly happened under such great care? I saw it one day, and it looked like someone had put a softball under his knee cap. Anyway, he ended up having surgery for a torn meniscus, and after two weeks of PT, he came back... to the same trainer. I know it's hard to believe. Just wait for the rest of the story. Being that the trainer was a certified specialist in corrective exercise, he knew exactly what to do from this point of the injury. He made the client step up on a box that was about eighteen inches high with all of his weight on his injured and recently operated-on knee. Sounds like a really smart thing to do. I went on about my business, trying to ignore the debauchery that was going on, and the next time I looked over at them, the client was lying down with an ice pack on his knee and his hands over his face, obviously in pain. What could have possibly gone wrong?

The guy could not walk because he had a knee the size of a cantaloupe, so paramedics had to carry him out. Stay tuned for next week's episode of *ER*. I felt bad for the guy, but he should have known after the first injury that his trainer was nothing but a quack. But this scenario goes on and on, and it wouldn't surprise me one bit to see that same guy working out again with the same trainer because his knee issues stemmed from something outside of their workouts, right? It's true people hurt themselves doing stupid things with their workouts all the time—they shouldn't but they do. But it's insult to injury when it's caused by a fitness instructor's incompetence. Exercise instructors hurt people all the time, and as always, it's put off as something the client did outside of their time with the trainer. Such a scam! Incompetence within the fitness instructor industry is as common as fitness equipment itself simply because most instructors have absolutely no idea what they're doing. And to make things worse, the so-called fitness evaluations they perform before they start working out their unfortunate clients are an absolute joke. Let's just call them what they really are: Fit-Less Evaluations.

Fit-Less Evaluations

For the most part, when a trainer begins working with a new client, the first thing they are supposed to do is a fitness evaluation and health history review. Yep, you guessed it: another big miss. They typically have the client step up and down on a bench for three minutes before checking their heart rate, taking a few measurements, and putting them through a stretch or two, and then off they go to the squat-a-thon and bicep bonanza. I've seen these so-called evaluations, and they're more like sales seminars where someone wins a TV at the end. By the way, did you know that almost all trainers who work for big gyms are paid according to how many training sessions they sell? I thought I'd throw that in there. So let's take a look at these fit-less evaluations and see exactly where these doctors—I mean trainers—fail the course.

Yes, No, or Maybe

Most of these evaluations are like speed dating. The trainer gets five minutes' worth of yes/no information from the new client and then off they go. I've seen it over and over again, and they make it look all official with their clipboards of generic questions they're supposed to ask, but it's mostly about obtaining the client's signature saying they won't sue in case of injury. The trainer might actually need that bit of information! The important stuff—like past injuries, joint issues, and other pre-existing health conditions—they'll figure those out as they go. Like when someone screams in pain or passes out from hypoglycemia—those are great indicators that something is wrong.

Push, Pull, and Get to Stepping

Push-ups, sit-ups, a sit and reach test, a three-minute step test, and maybe a plank comprise the typical evaluation lineup. Forget the old injuries; all of these tests are safe and for everyone. And that heart rate taken after that step test—what exactly will the trainer do with that? Nothing! They'll just tell their new victim to do cardio every day. Yep, more great advice from the heart of our fitness industry. And as far as modifying these tests for people with specific health issues, ha. Good luck with that one. That would take too much time and effort for the trainer, and there would not be enough time left in the hour to make the client really sore. Here's a good one: Let's see how much you can bench, squat, and curl.

Straight to Weights

A few sets of bench presses, a few lunges, some shoulder presses, a whole lot of abs, some bicep curls, and, of course, lots of good old squats are typically where these evaluations end up. There's nothing like making a new client sore after their first workout. You know, so they'll think they did some good and come back for more. And mixed in are the all-too-common questions most trainers ask new clients after a set of weights, such as, "Did you feel that?" "That burned, didn't it?" "Do you feel the pump?" and "Are you ready to get ripped, bro?" And the trainers always have their go-to exercise of standing on dumbbells to squat. Pretty complicated stuff here, so please don't feel intimidated.

Over Promising and Under Delivering

You can just imagine the rah-rah campaign that goes on with instructors and their clients. Encouragement is great, but a bunch of pumped up exaggerations and empty promises, or lies as I would call them, will come crashing down on the client when the body they were promised never materializes. There's an entirely different spin on this that I will talk about in Chapter 3 and again in Chapter 6, but for now, I'll leave it at that.

Realistic goals and expectations are great, but the misleading charades and fabricated appeasements to get clients to buy another ten-pack of training sessions and to keep them coming back is nothing short of FRAUD.

The Magical Disappearing Inches Act

Oh yes, the good old tape measure trick. It's very common for instructors to inflate a client's beginning measurements to give them a little "cushion" for when they measure again. And I still haven't figured out how you get accurate measurements when you take them over clothes, but trainers do it all the time. I guess I missed that one in my certifications as well. What about those body fat measurements? A couple of pinches, a little math, and presto! An instant and very inaccurate body fat assessment, which will be guaranteed to go down the next time it's measured. If you really want to know your true measurements, you're much better off doing them yourself.

Fit-less evaluations are mostly just that: quick, uneventful, and completely lacking in anything that's really useful and important to know about the client. Just so you will know, here is what a true fitness evaluation should look like:

Full and Complete Evaluation

Prior to Physical Testing:

- Liability waiver

- A complete review of the client's health, medication, and exercise history. If there is a history of health issues, a conversation

---

with their doctor is needed before doing any physical testing or working out. No doctoring here!

- Questions about their exercise preferences, work and home schedules, and any other scheduling issues

- Resting heart rates and blood pressure check

- Review client's goals, desires, and commitment level

- Review client's current eating plan

- Introduction to other workers and members and tour of the gym

Physical Testing:

- Slow to moderate warm-up while recording heart rates

- Stretching for all muscle groups

- Heart rate testing with bike, treadmill, or step

- Form and technique review

- Core assessment: a series of core exercises done very slowly on the ground, seated, and standing to assess muscular and skeletal imbalances and core flexibility

- According to client's personal health history, perform one set of ten reps with very light weight for each major muscle group. Only do body weight squats with no bar and no weights during testing. Use modifications for injuries or imbalances.

Post-Test Review and Program Design:

- Review with client any soreness or pain from evaluation.

- Provide a detailed explanation of suggested workout routine, including warm-ups, stretching, form and technique, resistance training, core training, and cardiovascular exercise.

- Review client's nutrition preferences and ask if they want nutritional guidance.

- Schedule client's exercise days and times.

- Encourage client to keep a journal.

There you go! It's not hard to do. It takes more time and attention to detail, but this is the only way to correctly perform a fitness evaluation. OK, enough of being serious. Let's move on to the fun stuff again. How about the actual workouts I see trainers putting their clients through? Oh yes, this is the good stuff!

Putting the Dumb in Dumbbells

Have you ever looked at a certain food at a low-end, all-you-can-eat buffet and wondered, "What the hell is that?" Or you see that vehicle driving down the road with duct tape and cardboard for a window, baling wire holding the bumper together, and two of the tires are those little bitty doughnuts, and you wonder, "How in the hell is that thing even on the road?" This is exactly what I think every day when I walk into the gym and watch trainers with their clients—cue the circus music again. It's almost always the same: way too much of one exercise, way too little of all the others, and a whole bunch of those weird made-up exercises to complete the show. Oh, and I can't forget the walking lunges with a barbell across the neck; this one seems to be the go-to exercise to really finish things off. Take a look at a few of these workouts and see if anything jumps out at you.

The Lunge-A-Thon: This is where a trainer has a client lunge around the gym for almost the entire session or a big part of it—most of the time with a barbell across the neck. Remember the camel and the knee ripper from earlier? This is the perfect place to see them both in action. The trainer might throw in a few other exercises, but the main goal is to lunge the client's legs off.

Multi-Station Monopoly: You know this one. This is where a trainer occupies several different machines for an extended period of time, or they will take several sets of dumbbells and barbells to an area of the gym where no one else can use them. I know people without a trainer who do this too, but a trainer should know better. Gyms get in on the monopoly game too by roping off certain areas and putting up signs that read For Personal Training Only. Believe me, you're better off staying out of this area altogether; the circus can get crazy.

The Counseling Session: Oh yes, the workout/counseling session. Trainers and their clients become close, but there is no need for a trainer to bring their personal life into their client's workout session. The client wants a workout, not a head case. Trainers need to leave their sad breakup stories out of their client's sessions and start concentrating on doing what the client paid them to do.

Seated Super Set: This one takes a lot of effort and concentration from the trainer. While the client is performing an exercise, the trainer counts the reps from a seated or lying position. Didn't you know that counting reps is very hard work? I mean, they can't be in beast mode the whole time they're in the gym.

The Three Ps: Also called the Push, Pull, and Puke, this is a very popular workout that trainers use to show their clients that they mean business. It usually includes a total body workout with very little rest, and, of course, squats are thrown in intermittently to get the desired puking effect. And if the client still hasn't lost their lunch, endless burpees and the lunge-a-thon should do the trick.

Like I said, the circus never closes, and if you want a front row seat, walk into the nearest gym and you're sure to get your money's worth. Just watch where you step; there's crap everywhere. Gyms full of bad trainers and exercise instructors are bad enough, but what about the countless overnight experts who post daily workout selfies on social media and offer their fitness coaching while you "Like" them? Is the advice they're offering any good, or do they just like seeing pictures of themselves?

Instant Coach—Just Add Selfie

From annoying open-mouth workout selfies to "ask me how" posts all over social media, a new breed of fit-less instructors are calling themselves "coaches" and offering to lend you their overnight expertise.

They'll post their annoying personal workout videos and pictures over and over again as well as their copied-and-pasted motivational quotes to try to make you think they really have their stuff together. Well, they don't. What really happened was they got involved in some kind of fitness company that sells workout videos, supplements, or diet plans, and they were given the "coach" title from the company itself, so this title has absolutely no merit at all. These so-called coaches are most likely pushing a bogus product as a "distributor" of some multi-level marketing (MLM) company, or they have joined a group promising you a body you can comfortably show off at the beach, but only if you use their products. In addition, these overnight coaches more than likely receive rewards through the company for posting workout videos, other ridiculous selfies, and selling products. Don't be fooled by their over-zealous smiles and happiness about their newfound health, and when they tell you they're a coach, ask them exactly how they became one. Chances are, you'll run into one of these overnight coaches in your gym, or if you're really unlucky, you'll get cornered by the Local Gym Workout Guru.

The Local Gym Workout Guru

You've seen them stalking around looking for the next opportunity to give exercise advice and talk your ear off. They'll tell you they either used to be a personal trainer or they still are, but they have another full-time job. And just like trainers, they'll throw around a few exercise terms and name a few key muscles, but you can almost guarantee that their advice is coming straight from some home-made exercise video they saw on the Internet, or it will be something they made up in their home gym. I'm talking about the local gym workout guru who is ready and willing to give you a spot, show you the best ways to up your bench, and give you an up-close demonstration of the latest YouTube workout they watched. I see this every day in the gym, but there's one instance that sticks out in my mind the most.

There was a young woman using a squat machine, and wouldn't you know, the workout guru walked over and started talking to her. I got closer to hear what he was saying, and as it turned out, she had a back injury and was told by her PT to use only machines for squats. The workout guru told her she could do regular squats if she did them right and that it would probably help her back. I didn't think she was going to listen but she did, and over to the squat rack they went. He, of course, showed her the "correct form," which was horrible and even had her jerking her hips forward at the top of the squat "to really strengthen her back," as he put it. I'll never forget it. It was on her third rep when she jerked at the top, screamed, and collapsed to the floor. It took her ten to fifteen minutes to stand up and walk out of the gym hunched over. Another victim of completely ridiculous exercise advice. The workout guru may look fit, but on the inside, they're a train wreck, just like their advice. Steer clear of them at all cost.

I've had my share of experiences with these guys, but I have a way of extinguishing them pretty fast. If you really want to avoid this person and get them to leave you alone, ask them the questions I provided at the beginning of this chapter, which should ward them off. But just in case you need more ammo, stare at their hairline when they talk to you, and tell them you can't do that exercise that way because you're allergic, and walk away. This should do it.

Fit-less instructors are indeed like politicians; they say
the right things and make promises of better times, but
when it comes time to deliver the goods, their true
colors are shady and their words turn into deceit.

Chances are, you may know a few personal trainers or fitness instructors, and you may even be one yourself, which means you're so close to the problem that you can't see it. As hard as it may be to believe the world of fitness instructors is really this bad, I can tell you from being on the front lines since 1990, it's a very upside-down, unhealthy industry. From teaching bad form and pushing pain, to playing doctor and double dipping with injuries, fitness instructors are the very core of the problem within an industry built on lies. So how does this happen? How is it that so many instructors get away with absurd and damaging ways of teaching exercises? It's really very simple. ANYONE can be a trainer or exercise instructor; it's just a matter of wearing workout clothes and having a business card. And those certifications most of them have? All they need is money, a computer, and to be able to read a little, and they're golden. Oh, those letters next to their names in their bios can look quite impressive, but when the lights come on, it's nothing but a certified ugly mess!

2 Bogus Credentials and Other Certified Crimes

Producing phony jewelry, purses, shoes, artwork, legal documents, and driver's licenses are all ways people can dupe us into buying something that's as fake and worthless as a three-dollar bill. Most retail stores have a pale green marker they run over bills of twenty dollars or more to make sure they're getting the real McCoy. And when it comes to coins, sports memorabilia, antiques, automobiles, and other popular items, there are reputable companies and experts who examine these items with a microscope to certify them as being either authentic and valuable, or authentic pieces of garbage. But when it comes to someone offering their fitness services and claiming to be certified, it's in your best interest to hit the brakes and take a closer look. Because at the end of the day, certifications don't mean a darn thing, and if you're not careful, you could end up losing an arm and a leg.

Having the word "certified" next to someone's name typically means they paid a fee, took a course, and upon passing an exam, became officially certified in their field of trade. Or in the case of becoming a certified fitness instructor, they paid a fee, took an online course at their leisure, had limitless chances to pass an open-book test, and became certified with a score of at least 70 percent. Yep, it's really that simple. And if they're willing to pay up and take several of these online courses from the same certification company, they will not only be super certified, they'll be an expert or master of their craft as well. After that, it's a simple matter of getting a business card and spreading the word that they're an officially certified personal trainer!

In this chapter, I'm going to show you why it doesn't take much more than a third-grade education to become a fitness instructor. In addition, I'll show you just how unfit many of these certification courses are and the really big pieces they're missing. What about the certification companies? Are they on the level, or have they found a way to cash in on a booming industry? And last, I'll give you my plan to make fit-less instructors either clean up their acts or hit the road to look for new jobs.

A License to Steal

Just like people, certifications come in all shapes and sizes; some are a lot easier going than others, some are more complicated, and some are just plain simple and uneventful. I will say that there are very few certification courses that do a great job making their students really learn the material. For the most part, if you can write your name and copy and paste answers, you're as good as certified. There's a certified fitness instructor everywhere you look these days, and if you look beyond the letters by a trainer's name, and see the embarrassing truth about how easy it is to become certified, you'll very quickly see why I call this whole certification business a certified crime.

> Basically, most certifications provide a license to steal—I'm talking about personal trainers taking clients' money without giving them anything worthwhile in return and robbing them of something much more valuable: their health.

So just how easy is it to get a fitness instructor certification? Just about as easy as opening a cereal box and digging around for the prize. The path to becoming a certified fitness instructor is paved with ease—so smooth and easy, even a baby could do it.

Baby Steps – The Path to Certification

- *Step 1:* Log in to a certification website, enter your personal information and your credit card number.

- *Step 2:* Read each chapter. Actually, you don't need to read anything; you can simply skip straight to the quizzes because everything is open book.

- *Step 3:* Take the open-book and un-timed quiz at the end of each chapter. Don't you worry now, you can take the quiz as many times as you want until you pass. And I mean no limits! Typically, the quizzes don't change if you have to keep taking them, so answers to these questions are learned, but as far as the application and understanding of the material, forget it.

- *Step 4:* After all chapters are read, take an open-book and un-timed final exam, which may or may not include a short essay. And if someone still finds this way too hard, they can actually Google the answers to most certification test questions and simply copy and paste. I'm not even kidding about this. And those essay / research sections of the exam? Knowing how to copy and paste will get you an easy A with these as well.

- *Step 5:* Submit your test answers.

- *Step 6*: Receive your test scores. If you failed, you have several attempts to retake the test and pass, for a small fee of course.

- *Step 7:* Receive your certification.

It's really this simple. And once someone has their certification in hand, they're like a teenager on the first day they get their driver's license; everyone should be expecting a wreck. As I said earlier, there are some certification courses that require you to be there in person for as long as a week, and their test is not an open-book format. But for the most part, the online version is what people go for, for obvious reasons. I've done both types, and the week-long, in-person courses are definitely more involved, but they all miss some very crucial components of teaching students how to be safe and effective fitness instructors. Take a look at what's missing in almost all certifications, and you'll see very quickly just how out of shape the whole certification thing really is.

Artificial Certifications – Why They're Worthless

Missing in Action

In all of the certification courses I've taken, there was little to nothing taught on correct form and technique in exercise. Most everyone else who was taking the course with me just flopped around and jerked their joints during the exercise demonstrations, just like the noncertified people I see. And did the instructor correct anyone? Absolutely not. In fact, there was never any discussion on how to perform exercises correctly. Oh, you get plenty of physiology review, but actual instruction on how to perform exercises the right way is, for the most part, nonexistent. You'll see pictures in your course book of people demonstrating certain exercises, and you'll almost learn which muscles are involved with each exercise, but the actual motion within each exercise is not discussed.

I remember my very first certification back in 1994, and man was I intimidated because everyone there had already gone through three or four other certification courses. Overhearing all of these experienced trainers discussing how long they had trained clients and how hard they had studied for this "very difficult" certification course almost made me get up and walk out before it started. I stayed, and I'm glad I did because when it came time to demonstrate correct form and technique on several exercises, I realized that I was surrounded by idiots. All of these people who had multiple certifications and who had been training people for several years were no more qualified to train someone than a drunk monkey. They were all horrible, and this was the very day I knew the fitness industry must be in really bad shape if these are the best of the best. I wasn't certified at the time and had only trained a few people at that point in my career, but I definitely knew wrong from right when it came to correct form and technique. That course was an absolute joke.

Over the next few years, I knew I needed to learn much more than what my first certification taught me, so I completed a physical therapy internship where I learned specific things about joint movement and joint health, and how to work with clients who have past or current injuries. Over the next twenty-some-odd years, I added a second PT internship, started working with doctors and surgeons, and to date I have designed fitness programs for more than seven thousand patients, and I've learned to work with almost every medical condition you can think of. I could not have learned these crucial and valuable lessons from taking all the certifications in the world because most of them do not address special health issues. There are a few specialized certifications that address special needs, but they are nowhere near enough for someone to truly learn what they need to know when training an individual with a serious health issue.

The Bigger Issues

The chances of a fitness instructor knowing how to safely and effectively train someone with a specific health condition like heart and cardiovascular problems, diabetes, joint pain, blood sugar issues, or lymphatic system problems are just about ZERO! Now think for a minute: What percent of our current population has one or more of these pre-existing health issues? Yep, at least 70–80 percent. And this is the same population that is most likely to seek out a fitness instructor to help them achieve better health. Do you see the problem? And like I stated in Chapter 1, most fitness instructors try to learn things as they go, and, unfortunately, their clients are the ones who pay the price. By the way, even the specialized certifications don't teach enough in this area; I know because I have several of them. Just like the other certifications, they teach plenty of physiology and supply information on fitness testing techniques, but they grossly miss many important variables. But because this ignorance is present from one end of the fitness industry to the other, nobody knows the difference anyway. I mean, who's going to report them?

Who's Watching Whom

Who's watching fitness instructors to make sure they are doing things right? Nobody! Even if we did have people watching them, the chances of the watchdogs recognizing right and wrong are slim to none. Can you say dumb and dumber? It's a free-for-all that allows instructors to train people any way they want because nobody knows the difference anyway.

Having a fitness instructor certification guarantees
good safe training just like a driver's license guarantees
good safe driving from a sixteen-year-old on day one.

Just hold your breath and hope nothing bad happens. I know trainers who have twice the certifications I have, but they are some of the worst trainers I've ever met. They're smart, in great shape, and have lively personalities, but the way they train their clients is nothing but detrimental and dumb. Here's another story of how a multi-certified personal trainer forever changed the life of a very unfortunate client:

> *This particular client was in his late sixties and had been working out with a personal trainer for about two weeks at this point. I had the chance to talk with this man one day while he was warming up, and through our conversation he informed me of his multiple back problems. These problems consisted of three herniated lumbar discs, spinal stenosis (narrowing of the spinal column), and a nasty case of sciatica. He stated he had been dealing with these conditions for the last three years and was trying to avoid surgery, and that's why he was using a personal trainer. I immediately thought, "Uh-oh, this isn't going to end well." For the next few days, I cringed watching this trainer—who was a certified corrective exercise specialist, by the way—make this man squat with a barbell on his back, do leg presses while letting his hips lift up, and (the killer) perform straight-leg deadlifts*

with, you guessed it, the humped back of a camel. Even my client was like, "WTH?" And then it happened. It was a quarter past ten on a Wednesday morning, and all of a sudden we heard someone yelling and moaning. And sure enough, it was the same gentleman. He was lying face down in a very crooked and bent way and was in excruciating pain. He ended up being rolled out on a gurney about thirty minutes later after the paramedics stabilized him; it was not a good sight at all. As it turns out, he had completely ruptured not one but three lumbar discs, had to have major back surgery, and I haven't seen him since. But his trainer is still there and going strong, breaking backs one client at a time. But he's specially certified and all, so it must have been just a freak accident, right?

This level of incompetence goes on every day in every gym, personal training studio, exercise class, and boot camp, and nobody knows the difference. Fitness instructors have zero accountability, and the artificial certifications they have don't help with this one bit. Certifications mean very little for several reasons; one of the biggest is that there are no prerequisites.

No Experience Needed

When I said a third-grader could pass a certification test and become a fitness instructor, I was serious. Most certification courses don't even require a high school diploma. If you can read and write, afford the fee, and can get in front of a computer, you're well on your way to becoming an artificially certified fitness instructor. Did I mention that there are no background checks either? That's right, a career felon can train you or your kids and you'd never know it. In the very gyms where I have trained over the course of my career, there were always three to four trainers with felony records working right beside me. What about those companies that give health coach titles to their followers who are preaching the graces of their wonder workouts and super supplements? Is this health coach title considered a type of certification, or is it given out like candy at Halloween to anyone in a costume?

Although fitness companies want you to think their health coaches are worthy of this designation, they are nowhere near deserving of being called coaches; they're much more suited for a title like Instagram cheerleader. In almost all cases, fitness companies require one thing for someone to be considered a coach: MONEY! All a person has to do is pay an up-front fee, pay a monthly fee, and push a little product. That's it, and it's off to the land of misleading and fake fitness advice. I've seen countless social media posts where these coaches offer fitness advice, and it always circles back to them pushing products to buy. Don't be fooled by companies claiming they have an endless supply of fitness coaches to help you reach your fitness goals; it's more about them reaching your wallet.

As far as I'm concerned, we might as well go ahead and put fitness instructor certifications in cereal and Cracker Jack boxes and toy vending machines, and maybe even use them as carnival prizes. They just aren't that valuable, especially when you're betting with not only your money but also your health. And that's exactly what people do when they hire a personal trainer, go to an exercise class, join a boot camp, or take advice from an overnight coach. They assume their health will improve if they follow their instructor's methods, but, as I hope you've learned by now, assuming your instructor's methods are safe can cost you a lot more than your gym membership. It could actually end up costing you an arm and a leg and a back and a...

In a *Doctor's Review* article, "Dangerous Personal Trainers," author Dimity McDowell stated, "Trainers don't need to meet any federal or state requirements. Even the woman who waxes your upper lip may have had more training—and she is certainly subject to more legal oversight—than the one who pushes your cardiovascular, muscular, and nervous systems, jacks up your heart rate and blood pressure, and strains your joints and ligaments."[2] This is a great association because it's funny and it's true.

What about certification companies themselves? Are some of them running rip-off rackets with overpriced "specialized certifications" and continuing education credits (CECs)? And at the same time, do they attempt to monopolize certification courses by requiring instructors to continually take *their* courses to keep certifications current? Take a look and see where certification companies might be faking the whole fitness thing too.

A Certified Rip-Off

For around $500, anyone can become a certified fitness instructor, and for another $500 every two years, they can stay certified. The certification business has evolved quite a bit over the last twenty years in terms of an increase in the actual number of companies and the different types of certifications offered. Some of these companies offer a vast menu of different certifications ranging from a basic certification course to extremely specialized courses in corrective exercises and youth instruction, but in most cases, much of the material is repetitive and grossly underachieving. I hear trainers and other fitness instructors telling potential clients that they have one or more of these specialized certifications, and they act as if they took a tough, grueling, and prestigious course. Like I said before, if you can read and write, you'll pass. Don't be fooled by someone who flashes a specialized certification to justify their ability to teach fitness; it just doesn't carry any weight; pun intended. What about the CECs required by certification companies? Are they valuable, and do they keep a fitness instructor truly up-to-date on correct exercise? Or are they overpriced and just another way for the company to create revenue for itself?

CEC or Continued Waste of Time

Overall, I feel CECs are definitely needed in most careers, but I also feel certification companies take great advantage of this by requiring CEC courses too often and overcharging at the same time. Most, if not all, fitness certification companies make it mandatory for their students to take CEC courses every two years to maintain their certification status. From my experience in these courses and the fact that it doesn't seem to help the current incompetency level of the trainers I've seen, I feel these CEC courses are inept and required too often. You might ask, "If trainers are really that bad, doesn't it make sense to require them to take more classes so they can learn correct ways of exercise?" This is a great question, but when the certification courses themselves are already not fit for their purpose, you can probably guess how little these trainers will learn from a CEC course from the same company. And taking enough CEC courses to obtain the required number of hours ends up being comparable to a new certification course in terms of expense. Could this be something companies do on purpose to keep fitness instructors taking their courses instead of another company's courses?

You're Stuck with Us

Certification companies typically require CEC hours every two years in order to keep certifications current and active. To keep things easy and "convenient" for their students, companies have a whole menu of CEC courses from which to choose to keep certifications active. The thing is, once you add up the cost of taking enough CEC courses to satisfy their requirements, you can just about take an entirely new certification course for the same cost. And wouldn't you know it, this one course satisfies the entire CEC credits needed to stay current. And since it's typical for a company to accept only certain CEC courses, it incentivizes instructors to stick with certain companies in order to stay current. I did it. I have taken several certification courses from the same company, simply because of convenience and cost. Overall, I feel certification companies take advantage and cash in by requiring too many CECs too often when most of these courses are not worth anywhere near what the certification companies are charging. Yet another problem in the fitness industry that is camouflaging itself as something healthy.

So how do we fix this mess? I'm going to go ahead and tell you that state and federal regulation of fitness instructors won't change a thing. Neither will a licensing requirement or stricter and more involved certification courses. Even if you implemented all of these things, it would be impossible to monitor all instructors to make sure they are teaching safe exercise methods. Oh, it would definitely create more money for the state and other regulatory agencies, but the problem of incompetent instructors would be untouched. OK, so what's the answer? Fortunately, the blueprint already exists. We do what sports teams, companies, and the business of politics all do when something within their organization goes horribly awry and they need a big change. They get rid of the dead weight, clean house, or cut bait, all of which mean getting rid of the people causing a stink and getting a fresh start. Sounds pretty good to me, but since we are talking about the fitness industry, let's call it Trimming the Fat.

Trimming the Fat

I'm going to give you four suggestions we can all do to get rid of that unwanted weight that has attached itself throughout the fitness industry. Take a look and see my plan for sweating out the bad guys, burning up the bad fat, and cleaning up a dirty industry.

Idiot Alert

Take what I have shown you over these first two chapters and use it to recognize bad instructors; it'll be easy because they're everywhere. While you're at it, share this information with someone else so they can have their idiot radar on as well. It has to start with this because if this idiotic behavior isn't recognized, it will never stop. Just look for the crazy stuff I showed you in Chapter 1 and you'll see it with no problem. If you're currently using a personal trainer or taking a group class, remember those four questions to ask, and look for the camel, the turbo lifting, and the lumbar leveler; they're in every gym, every single day. Spend some time watching the circus acts going on with clients and their trainers. You might as well; it's a free show. Last, if you or someone else is using a trainer or taking an exercise class and the instructor advises you to "work through the pain," the instructor is a certified idiot; leave while you can. Now, if you've hired a trainer to work with your kid, or your kiddo is involved in any kind of group exercise, a different approach is definitely needed.

No-Kid Zone

Talk about a disaster waiting to happen! Putting your kid's health in the hands of a personal trainer is asking for trouble. I know it sounds like a great idea and a way for your kiddo to get some good exercise activity or to get ahead in their game, but the risk of injury is imminent. This one really gets under my skin because the kid is going to do everything the trainer asks, even if it's painful.

> I can't tell you how many times I've watched a kid grabbing their shoulder, rubbing their lower back, or limping through the gym while their trainer tells them, "Keep going! No pain, no gain!"

Again, stupidity at its finest and a complete disregard for health. Here's what you can do: The next time your kid has a session with a trainer or is part of an exercise group, sit in on the session and watch very closely. Don't be afraid to ask questions, and get the instructor to explain things like I mentioned at the beginning of Chapter 1. Instructors have to be called out, put on the spot, held accountable, and made to explain exactly what they're doing and why they're having your child do certain exercises. And like I said earlier, don't accept vague, evasive answers. Make them give you specifics, and don't let them off until they do. Better yet, keep your kid away from them and avoid the whole thing. Be sure to ask your kid if they have any pain during or after their workouts, and if they do, pull them out and have a little visit with the instructor. It might not even be a bad idea to consult with an attorney as well. Now we're getting somewhere.

Bring on the Lawsuits

Instead of chasing ambulances, attorneys should hang out in gyms and around boot camps and give out business cards; what an absolute gold mine! I'm always surprised there aren't more lawsuits filed in the fitness industry. Maybe it's the attorneys I need to educate on the high level of fraudulent activity within the fitness industry. I'd even help them make a commercial about it. Can you picture what that would look like? Here's the perfect commercial: Hi, I'm attorney _____ _____. Has your fitness instructor put you through the camel, the lumbar leveler, or the rotator ripper? Do you have increased joint pain from your workouts? Do you have trouble walking after a killer leg day? If so, don't wait another minute. Call us NOW! Call 1-800-BAD-TRAINER, and let the real workout begin!

Remember the PPP workout? The push, pull, and puke? That would be a commercial highlight for sure. The lawsuits are there, folks; it's just a matter of getting people to file them. If anyone ever needs an expert witness for a fitness instructor lawsuit, I'm in! Now what about this certified mess? How do we fix it?

Fit to be Certified

In addition to improving the content of instructor certification courses, we can add much more stringent requirements, which will weed out the bad instructors. First of all, physical therapy internships must be required before any certification is given. I'm talking about requiring a six-month to one-year internship working with people who have injuries before anyone is allowed to train others. And the physical therapist has to approve and release the trainer to begin a fitness career. Second, every fitness instructor should have to both demonstrate and explain correct form and technique on a variety of exercises, including modifications for health issues, in front of a panel of physical therapists and orthopedic surgeons before receiving their certification. This should have to be repeated every two years to keep their certifications active. How's that for

CECs? And last, before any certification is given, every applicant should be subject to a background check, and the status of this check should be on the certification itself—kind of like the restrictions on a driver's license. I guarantee you this: If these changes in certification requirements were adopted, there would be a whole lot fewer fit-less instructors running around busting joints, except their own of course.

As you can see, most fitness instructor certifications aren't worth the paper on which they're printed. It's because anyone with half a brain can get one, most are void of crucial material, and once someone becomes certified, there's absolutely no accountability they're going to teach safe and productive exercise. I wasn't kidding when I said the circus was in town and you can get front row seats in any gym or boot camp. I've almost resorted to wearing blinders when I go to the gym so I don't have to see the clown acts. But no matter what I do to ignore the fact that our fitness industry is full of very bad instructors, there are several reminders in every gym waiting to show me their juggling and balancing acts.

> From the low fitness IQ most trainers have and the circus acts they call workouts, to the dysfunctional and missing content of many certification courses, the fitness instructor industry is mostly a monkey see, monkey do playground where YouTube workouts rule, and just about anything goes.

Fitness instructors are pretty good at making people think they're on top of their game and that they have all the answers to any fitness woes, but the BS detector is working overtime and getting really overheated by the squat rack.

So there you have it—two chapters full of fake fitness to get this party started. Now what? Oh yes, the best is yet to come. There's a whole other part of the fitness industry that definitely looks the part and is ready and willing to show you how to really put on a show. They'll swear up and down that their amazing and completely unnatural looking physiques are nothing but products of long hard hours in the gym and precise nutrition. And that little pharmacy tucked down deep in their gym bag or hidden away at home contains nothing but all-natural supplements and vitamins. Right! Just like those needles they have are for sewing.

3 Real Muscle or Just Flex Appeal?

Can you imagine what the fitness industry would look like without drugs? It's actually kind of funny if you think about it. I can tell you the world of bodybuilding would look a lot different; they'd all be two to three times smaller and actually look somewhat natural, but at least they'd still have nice fake tans. What about the women's bikini, fitness, figure, and physique competitions? Would they look different too? You bet they would! And that extra postorbital growth (protruding lower forehead), outrageous hip-to-waist ratio, and well-defined jawline would all be things of the past. What about those who excel in other fitness sports like triathlons, weight lifting/tire flipping/aerobic contests, mixed martial arts (MMA), and boxing? How badass would they be without their muscle dope? I'm willing to bet they wouldn't be half the athlete or half the size without it. We can't forget fitness models; they have as much reason to juice up as anyone else. Do you think they take part in the roid ritual to get their fit look? And what about the jacked-up people walking around in gyms getting their swole on with their year-round vascularity, 6 percent body fat, and arms as big as most people's legs? Would they be nearly as muscular and ripped without their pharmaceutical aids? That's a guaranteed no. And last, what about the countless other people walking around with testosterone prescriptions and the surge of the miraculous time-machine transformations of the forty- to sixty-year-olds with twenty-year-old bodies? Are they on something too? Yes, they are, but it's all OK because their doctor says so.

The problem isn't that these people are taking steroids and other drugs, it's that most of them lie about doing it at the expense of others who think they can look the same way with nothing but exercise, clean eating, and a gallon jug of amino acids.

It's all just another gym bag full of pumped-up lies from our "fitness" industry, and once you read through this chapter, you'll see why the "battle of the bulge" is nothing but a raging roid battle of who can mix up the best bottle of magic muscle in the chemistry lab. Although a few of the groups taking steroids are obvious to most people, there are a few groups who will surprise you. Let's just say females aren't so full of sugar and spice after all as they do their best to turn that X chromosome into a Y. What about sixty becoming the new twenty? Is our aging population getting in on the "stick" too? Yes, they are, and most of them are lying about it just like everybody else. To really beef up this chapter, I'm also going to tell you bizarre and unbelievable stories from personally witnessing the rise and fall of one of the biggest steroid rings ever, which ended with the penitentiary for some and, unfortunately, the grave for others.

> The fitness industry has given "juicing" and "cycling"
> entirely new meanings that have absolutely nothing to
> do with blenders or bikes.

So who's on the stuff? A lot more people than you may think. Let's take a look at everyone who is using steroid cocktails and fat-be-gone drugs to increase their flex appeal. The perfect place to start is at the top of the steroid society with the biggest group of roid wranglers of all: bodybuilders.

The Steroid Society

Bodybuilding

Back in 1990, when I first started my personal trainer career, I was surrounded by some of the biggest men and women I'd ever known—and I mean huge! There was a Mr. USA, several who had been crowned either Mr. or Mrs. Texas, and many others who looked like walking bags of boulders with tans. And those women were almost as big as the guys, walking around with rapidly diminishing thyroids, superhero jaws, and voices as deep as mine. And, of course, all of these huge people were personal trainers using their bodies as walking billboards. But just like most advertisements, it's what they're not telling you that discredits their promises. Today, I know many bodybuilders, and although most of them are nice enough, there's always that cult-like, cliquish, and secretive air about them. They don't know it, but I can see right through them and their quiet conversations over in the corner, their amazing transformations in a matter of weeks, and how their teenage acne problems seem to have somehow re-emerged on their backs and shoulders. Again, this book isn't about the harmful side effects of taking steroids, nor is it about taking steroids in general; it's about how a lot of people lie about the fact that they take drugs to get that lean, hard, and fit body they have, and then convince others they can do the same with only exercise and eating healthy. And bodybuilders are among the worst at it.

Saying that the world of bodybuilding is super competitive is an understatement. And it's not so much about who trains the hardest and has the best diet; it's more about who has access to the best chemist.

Look, at least 90–95 percent of them take steroids, and this is probably a conservative number. There's just no way these guys can get this big or compete without steroids. It's fair to say that I cannot prove the number is this high, but after witnessing it for myself over the last 27 years and counting, interviewing bodybuilders, and researching bodybuilding and steroid websites, all arrows point to this high number.

According to a 2017 *Bodybuilding.com* article, "30 Lies of Bodybuilding," the number one lie is "You can get as big as a pro bodybuilder without taking steroids; it just takes longer." The article also said, "Despite what many of the magazines say, all professional bodybuilders use either steroids or steroids in combination with other growth-enhancing drugs. Without manipulating hormones, it just isn't possible to get that degree of muscularity, the paper-thin skin, and the continuing ability to pack on mass . . ."[3] This echoes what I consistently found in my interviews and from my research on other websites.

And those "all-natural" contests you see advertised: more bull. There's no such thing. As you'll see in Chapter 5, there are all kinds of ways to fake the pee and get around the so-called testing in these contests. There are countless websites, articles, videos, and magazines that specialize in exactly what drugs to take, how much to take, and when to take them. Actually, several of these sites claim they can get the drugs for you as well; whether they're the real thing or not is another subject. Absolutely crazy! Information about "how to" when it comes to taking drugs is unlimited, but it's the balls to admit they're doing it that are lacking, and I mean literally. Or in the case of female users, it's the lack of... well, considering the side effects, you could say the same thing. They don't have balls, but something else is definitely growing there; let's just say it looks like a miniature penis.

What about bodybuilders who are personal trainers? I mean, damn; they've got the look, right? So it makes sense that most anyone would want them as a trainer. But sooner or later, one or more things happen, and it's all a matter of time before everything loses its pump and comes crashing down. Take a look at the three most common outcomes of using a personal trainer who has a part-time job as a walking pharmacist.

Personal Trainer or Personal Pharmacy?

Empty Promises

I've seen this more times than I can count. You'll see a body-builder/trainer with a brand-new client and after about a month, the client starts asking many questions about why they aren't seeing any progress. And with these questions come outrageous answers from the trainer (see Chapter 1). This buys some time, but eventually the client's number of training sessions starts to dwindle and then they're gone. This is a great example of how the look of a bodybuilder alone can get them unlimited personal training clients, and that's not a good thing. If a client sticks around for an extended time with their new super-built trainer, it's only a matter of time before the real pain shows up and they have to trade in their training dues for insurance deductibles.

The Injury from Hell

This one can get bad! You'll see bodybuilders pushing their clients to train just like they do with never-ending sets and reps, huge volumes of different exercises, and training until they puke— grunting and groaning optional. This is how most bodybuilders train because the steroids and other drugs they're taking help them recuperate much quicker than a normal person, which allows them to work out much harder than everyone else. But when they apply this same training method to someone who isn't taking steroids, it always ends badly.

> I've seen torn pecs, torn cartilage, complete muscle
> separation from the bone, broken bones, and many
> other injuries from bodybuilders training their clients
> like they're on the special sauce too.

I can't believe some of these clients stick around even after a major injury. Maybe it's because there's another offer waiting behind door number three at which they'd like to take a peek. Yep, you guessed it; the opportunity to take the exact same "supplements" their trainer is taking.

Get with the Program

This is the worst one of all. You can always tell when it happens because all of a sudden, a client starts to make incredible gains of strength and muscle, experience a substantial loss in body fat, and sprout a back full of acne. They'll start making this super-fast progress and just like their trainer, they'll lie and say it's from their hardcore training and diet. Same old story; same old bull. You can also tell when the client runs out of money because all of that new muscle they found disappears once their steroid fund dries up. Speaking of drying up, they may have gotten scared because, although their muscles grew, there were other body parts that not only shrank, but also stopped working for the most part. Yep, that's a bad sign. BBs for balls and a little smokie that just can't get the job done.

It's the "flex appeal" that makes bodybuilding and personal training go hand-in-hand. These trainers look like they have it all figured out so why wouldn't someone want to train with them? Like I said previously, when a bodybuilder trains a client, it always plays out in one of three ways, all of which inevitably leave the client with the short end of the stick. From what I've witnessed since I entered this business, steroids have a way of taking over not only the body, but also the mind. I've seen bodybuilders really lose it with their clients, get really mad at other trainers who were using a piece of equipment they needed, and get furious when someone simply walks in between them and a mirror while they were doing an exercise. These minor outbursts are all really common and more annoying than serious, but I've also seen trainers completely blow their lids. Back in the early '90s, I had the unfortunate experience of getting caught up in the worst roid rage I'd ever seen, and it went like this:

This story I'm about to tell you may seem completely out there and unbelievable; that's because that's exactly what it was.

> *It was five o'clock on a weekday, and I had just started a session with my client when all of a sudden, a really big guy, about five nine, 240 pounds, started screaming, "I am God," as loud as he could right in the middle of the gym. I was like, "WTH?" And everyone else in the gym got quiet. The really big guy was with his brother, and you could tell that his brother was trying to calm him down and get him out of the gym. There were several times when it looked like the two of them were about to fight. This went on for about five minutes and then it escalated.*

> *This guy started walking up to different people who were working out and yelling, "I am God," and flexing like he was a pissed off gorilla in his cage. I even looked at a good friend of mine who was training right beside me and told him we were going to have to do something, so be ready.*

> *After about two or three minutes of this, the brother had managed to get the big guy to the front of the gym (this was at five o'clock on a weekday so the gym was full). This is where the real rage began, and I've never seen anything like it in my life. This man picked up his brother, who was even bigger than he was, lifted him over his head and body slammed him onto the concrete gym floor. As his brother lay on the floor in pain, I waited for this guy to turn his back to me, and I ran as fast as I could and tackled him from behind. Boy was he pissed! He started to lift me up like I was nothing, and thank the lord, five other guys came in to help. It took all six of us to hold this guy down, and with all of my weight on his one arm he was still lifting me completely off the ground. I looked over and he was doing the same thing with his other arm. After about two minutes of all of us*

struggling to restrain him, he started having a grand mal seizure, so we had to get off of him.

As he was having this seizure, the paramedics came through the door and started their assessment. One looked up and asked everyone there, "What's this guy on?" Neither his brother nor anyone else said a word, and then the paramedic repeated, "It's a matter of life and death; what's he on?" His brother finally came clean. He named three or four different steroids, including GHB (gamma hydroxybutyrate, also known as liquid ecstasy), an anti-depressant, and a heart medication. About a minute later, this guy regained consciousness, and the fight was on again! He tried to get up, and I'll never forget his eyes; he looked like he was ready to kill every-one there, and he was yelling again that he was God.

That's when the cops got there, and as they watched us struggle to hold him down, they immediately called for back-up—they were nervous too. Once three other cops got there it took nine guys to lift him up on the gurney, and once he was there, the cops double handcuffed each arm to the rails, tied six belts around his body, and wheeled him out. And as he was headed out the door, he was still yelling, "I am God," and was also yelling that he was going to kill everyone in there, including the cops.

That was a bad day, and guess what? About a month later, he did the same thing at another gym. After this happened, all of the body-builders, fitness pageant contestants, and the other really big and fit people in this particular gym stayed silent about the incident, and for some reason, they all seemed pretty nervous for a while. I wonder why? This is when things started to really go downhill, but I'll save that story for later.

Bodybuilders are just one group that is trapezius-deep in steroids; there are plenty of others to talk about, and this next group is one that surprises most people.

Typically, when people think of steroid use, it's the
huge hulking guys they envision, right?

But there's a whole other group you wouldn't expect that is trading in manicures for muscle and tiaras for testosterone. I'm talking about women. That's right! The world of bikini, figure, fitness, and physique contests is full of bulked-up beauties parading around their unbelievably lean, hard bodies and claiming it is all because of their killer workouts and chicken and broccoli diets. Insert that BS word here again because just like with bodybuilding, 90–95 percent of these women have the testosterone of a twenty-year-old male, and the chins, foreheads, night sweats, and anxiety to prove it.

Girls Gone Wild

I have to admit, I was naïve about steroid use by females until about twelve years ago. I got to know a few women who competed in female fitness events, and they told me in great detail the amount and types of steroids and other drugs that are used by most of these competitors. They showed me before and after pictures of their steroid use and the difference was astounding. They even pointed out the difference in their facial features, which had definitely become more masculine. One woman even said that her before and after pictures looked like a brother and sister; that's exactly what I thought but I didn't want to say anything.

Over the course of a month, I interviewed twenty-three female fitness contestants and I asked every one of them, "How many women in these contests take steroids and other drugs?" Every single one of them answered, "All of us take drugs. There's no way to compete if you don't do drugs." There were a few who just froze when I asked them, but it didn't take them long to come clean. Most of these young women also told me they experienced severe anxiety, serious hormone disruption, and depression while taking these drugs, but accepted these side effects as trade-offs for their fake physiques.

I also asked them, "Was it worth it? Are you going to keep taking steroids or get away from the whole thing?" Most of them responded by saying they would probably take just enough drugs to keep them looking fit so they can keep competing in contests and building their personal training business, or for aesthetic reasons with other careers such as professional cheerleading, dancing, and so on. I then asked them the burning question: "Do you think it's right to mislead and lie to your personal training clients or customers by not telling them you take drugs to get your fit looking body?" Their answer: "I don't really feel bad because everyone else is doing it too, so why can't I?" My answer: "You're exactly right; everyone else is doing it. But you're also dead wrong to take advantage, mislead, and lie to people; that's fraud. And by the way, I don't take drugs, and my business is booming and has been for twenty-seven years." Their response? Silence!

With female fitness contestants, it's not so much about who works out the hardest and eats the cleanest; it's more about the quality of what's coming through the needle.

Don't let the titles of these contests fool you; almost all of the contestants are on the juice, and it's been this way for decades. In the 2001 *ThinkSteroids.com* article, "D-Cups and D-Bol—Women and Anabolic Steroids," author Anthony Roberts wrote about the high levels of Anavar, Winstrol, Clenbuterol, and growth hormones that he had knowledge of female fitness competitors using.[4] Again, although the proof of such high usage of steroids by female competitors is hard to substantiate without dropping in on them unannounced and testing them, all the signs are pointing in the same direction, just like the needles they use.

Another thing to remember is that not all steroids and drugs are for gaining huge amounts of muscle; there are several types designed to make you keep your muscle while you lose your body fat and water. In Chapter 4, I'm going to show you exactly what drugs are being taken all across the fitness industry, and when you see what these drugs do, you'll definitely start to connect the dots with these female contestants. If you're like me, you may not fully understand the differences between the many different women's contests, so I have listed them here with some short descriptions for each one.

Bikini

The bikini division is known for its model walk presentation on stage. This division focuses on balance and shape as well as overall physical appearance. Complexion, skin tone, poise, and overall presentation are all taken into consideration. This category typically has the largest number of entries, and the competition is very high. The key words here are "competition is very high," which is more than enough reason for these women to resort to steroids to get a leg up. Like I said earlier, not all steroids are for gaining huge amounts of muscle; some are just for leaning out, and contestants take them by the handfuls. And if they aren't taking steroids, there's a very high likelihood they are taking other types of illegal drugs that burn body fat like butter in a frying pan. Now, let's look at the next level up.

Fitness

This is known for being the division involving an aerobics, dance, and gymnastics performance. This routine is judged based on the accuracy and difficulty of showing strength, flexibility, cardiovascular endurance, and a solid overall presentation. Judges score the competitors' bodies according to firmness, symmetry, proportion, and overall physical appearance. Remember, steroids aren't only for the look of leaner and harder bodies; they also help improve athletic performance. Again, even more reasons for these women to get on the juice. This next level of competition is where things really start to get interesting.

Figure

It's in these contests where the amount of muscle a woman has starts to be a big factor. Figure competitors are known for muscle tone and symmetry, and less focus is placed on muscle size in comparison to bodybuilding. However, judges do look for a greater amount of muscularity in the physical appearance and muscle tone. The ideal figure competitor has muscle tone throughout the body, shapely lines, and firmness, but is not excessively lean. The key thing here is that judges look for muscularity and muscle tone, which leads to a greater reason to get a little help from the steroids. It's also during these contests where the contestants even stand and pose just like bodybuilders. Again, most of these contests claim to be all natural, but as you'll soon find out, there is no such thing.

Physique

Physique is a division that focuses on symmetry, shape, proportion, muscle tone, poise, and beauty flow. This is one size down from bodybuilding; contestants are encouraged to avoid certain bodybuilding qualities such as being shredded, ripped, or vascular, but most end up like that anyway. Physique competitors should have the overall look found in figure, with a little more muscularity. Several articles I read categorize this class of competition as being one step below bodybuilding, and if you research this type of contest, you'll see why. And if a woman really wants to blow things out, she can take one more step up and compete with the really big bodies.

Female Bodybuilding

Yeah, it's all natural; can't you tell? From what I have read in my research, female bodybuilding is losing its drive, and the number of contestants is dropping by the year, but it still has enough juice to stay alive. I also researched exactly which kinds of steroids these women take to get their massive amounts of muscle and it blew me away. I cover this in more detail in the next chapter, but let's just say it can be as much as the male bodybuilders take. It's OK, take all you want ladies; just be honest when someone asks you how you got that big. Or just talk a little bit, and they'll figure it out from your new voice and all.

As you can see, the level of muscularity required for these different contests increases, starting with the bikini and going all the way through to the bodybuilding competitions. Therefore, the need for instant lean muscle is indeed high, and many will stop at nothing to get their fill. As I researched this, I found many articles comparing the figure and physique competitions to that of lower level bodybuilding because of the unnatural amounts of lean muscle most of these females possess. And what's even more interesting is the number of articles and blogs describing in great detail the specific kinds of steroids and drugs, the amount, and the steroid cycles that are most popular for women within these types of competitions. To take things even further, there are countless articles that break down the exact dosage per day and how to pass the drug test before the competition.

Yes, women are in on it too, and just like all the other steroid users, they lie about it as much or more than anyone. So if you're a female and you look at these female contestants with envy and wonder why you can't look like they do, even with all of your working out and eating right, just know that their world of fake fitness will eventually come crashing down, and their thyroid will be crashing with it—all while you remain fit as a fiddle. So what about the other kinds of fitness sports? Are they jumping on the roid wagon and artificially beefing up as well?

From Pros to Joes

From professional sports like football and baseball, to the grueling endurance of a triathlon, to the "who can drop a barbell from over their head and make the most noise" contests, people are pushing, pulling, jumping, running, and lifting their bodies to new limits on a daily basis. And again, onlookers at these events are mostly under the impression that all of these participants are able to do what they do and look the way they do solely from intense exercise and strict eating. Where's my bullhorn? Bullsh*t alert! The truth is, steroid use in these sports and many others is probably as common as it is in bodybuilding and women's fitness contests. Why? Because with the exception of professional football and baseball, most of these sports are all under the radar. I mean, who would think a cyclist, a runner, a volleyball player, or a tennis player would need to take steroids? But they do, and they've been caught. But they all have their excuses: "It was only a cream for my arthritis," "I didn't know it was illegal," "It was prescribed by my doctor for my ADD," "I thought it was just vitamins," and "I was told it was only for energy," to name a few. And here we go again with the lies. Even when they're caught, they still act like they had no idea they were taking steroids. Believe me, they knew damn well what they were taking. Take all you want, just grow some balls and tell people the truth: Your newfound muscle and immense improvement on the field is fake.

There are all kinds of fitness sports that go unmentioned when it comes to taking steroids mostly because these types of sports typically aren't associated with steroid use. But they're out there, and there are plenty of participants who fake their way through the ranks with their roid regimen, just like players in professional football and baseball do. Can you imagine a chess player, a badminton player, or a debate team member taking steroids? I'd probably watch that. Let's start at the top of the sports world and work our way through these different fitness sports and see how all of them have juiced up their game; you're going to be very surprised at some of these.

Professional Baseball and Football

This one is no great secret. I'm sure all of us are well aware of the huge baseball steroid scandal which alleged drug use by many popular players, such as Barry Bonds, Mark McGwire, Alex Rodriguez, Jose Conseco, Rafael Palmeiro, Ryan Braun, and many others. It was really obvious because some of these guys all of a sudden looked like bodybuilders in baseball uniforms—and in a very short amount of time. But hey, they were just working out a lot, eating healthy, and using a cream to help with their soreness. Many players were busted after Biogenesis Labs Inc. handed over patient documents, and what do you know, it was like Christmas for the Major League Baseball (MLB) investigators as a huge number of players were exposed. It was even uncovered that many of these players started taking steroids as early as high school. No surprise there either. Even though baseball is the sport most known for steroids and performance enhancing drugs (PEDs), professional football has a black eye too, and since the early '90s several players were suspended for PED use. If you ask me, most of these players, along with thousands of others, got their steroid start many years earlier in high school and college. I'm not going to use any statistics on steroid use here because they're worthless, simply because most users aren't honest about it, and there are many ways to fake a steroid test—we'll talk about this in Chapter 5. Professional baseball and football aren't the only professional sports injecting the juice; sports like tennis, boxing, MMA, and others are doing the deceiving drug dance as well.

The Other Sports

Athletes in sports like tennis, volleyball, soccer, and triathlons don't test positive for steroid use for two main reasons: The testing is very rarely done, and it's done during the competition. Most blood doping and steroid use takes place during an athlete's training, and they can get off the juice in time to show a clean test result. Oh, it's there, but it's almost like these other sports don't want to catch anyone doing it. Remember when Lance Armstrong got busted? How many people were shocked at that? I've said this before, and I'll say it again: Some steroids and other "fitness" drugs won't add muscle, they'll simply allow you to recuperate quicker so you can train harder.

Just like with women's fitness contests, don't be fooled
by the type of sport or how the athlete looks; steroid
use is everywhere, and the lies are right there with it.

Speaking of fake fitness, over the last several years I've watched one particular method of exercise grow to one of the most popular fitness sports ever, and when I see the way these people look in these contests, I just shake my head and wonder what their dosages are and how much their joint replacements are going to cost. They sure act tough as they grunt, groan, and throw barbells, tires, and other weights around, but if you would take away their roids, their muscular bodies and crazy strength would go away, and their fitness boasting would surely die a very fast death too.

Here's a rule of thumb you can use when it comes to steroid use and sports: If there is competition, there will be steroid use, and as the level of competition increases, so will the use of steroids. You can't deem any sport immune to steroid use, even the ones you absolutely would never associate with steroids.

Even in the most obscure and under-the-radar sports, steroids and other banned drugs have found their way into numerous athletes' game plans. It makes you think a little more about sports like beach volleyball, soccer, archery, and even bowling as having athletes who take steroids. I know it's crazy, but I guarantee you a few tests would turn up positive if they tested these athletes too. What about fitness transformation contests you see advertised everywhere—are some of the contestants running on roids too? Oh yes, the drugs are running fast and furious baby, and if you take enough of them, you might just win yourself a brand-new TV!

Roid-Rigged

Fitness transformation contests are everywhere, especially within gyms, in boot camps, and online, and I bet you there's not a hint of steroid testing either. As small as most of these contests are, I've seen the steroid users rise up, come riding in on their stair steppers, and take first place. Just the other day I was in a gym that holds these contests on a regular basis and right beside me there were two guys and one girl talking in great detail about their current "stack" of steroids. And wouldn't you know it, all three of them were in the contest. There is no level of competition too small for steroids, and these fitness transformations are not immune. I've seen some of the before and after pictures on the advertisements for these contests, and they look like cartoons to me. And it's funny how the word "natural" seems to be written in big letters like it's a guarantee or something. Here's what I say: Let's include blood, urine, and lie detector tests with these transformation contests and see just how many people back out before it even starts. OK, I think I've beaten these people up enough. Who's next? Oh yes, the world of fitness models. Hey, look at me! If you buy this product and start with it immediately, you can look just like me in only a few weeks. And there goes the BS alarm again.

Fitness Models

Believe me, makeup, great lighting, exercise, and a good diet aren't the only things that make these models look awesome. Yep, many of them are walking the runway to the roid round-up; they're just harder to spot. *Nattyornot.com* had this to say about fitness models and drug use: "Unfortunately, professional fitness is neither as healthy nor as pure as the industry claims. Just like competitive bodybuilders, the leading fitness models are on the juice, and the whole industry is full of back stabs, lies, and deceptions. Undoubtedly, modern fitness models inject steroids."[5]

The difference between many fitness models and those who compete in bodybuilding and fitness pageants is basically nothing but the dosage. As I said earlier, not all steroids and drugs are going to make you big and muscular; there are many designed to keep you lean with low body fat while maintaining your muscle. Because the competition among fitness models is just as high as it is among bodybuilders and other fitness contestants, the pressure to have the perfect look is indeed high. Do you think fitness models are tested for steroids? Ha! No way. Companies don't give a rat's a** what models take as long as they look good. If a model is in a commercial for a piece of fitness equipment, an exercise program, or a brand-new wonder supplement, they have to look the part. I'll get into more detail about fitness advertisements in Chapter 6, but for now, let's stick to how these fitness models fake their fit.

As I was doing my research for this chapter, I ran across several fitness model forums, and out of curiosity, I logged in and started reading through several conversation threads. Although I expected to see a few conversations about steroids and other drug use, I was not expecting what I found. At least 90 percent of the conversations were about how, what, and when to take certain drugs leading up to a photo or commercial shoot. It was truly unbelievable! And these weren't average dialogues; these were specifically outlining exactly how much of each drug to take, when to take them, how to stack several specific drugs together, and how to avoid getting caught. And to top things off, many of these conversations included people saying, "Where can I get these drugs?" and "Private message me," all of which more than likely led to more explicit conversations about buying and using steroids. The biggest thing I got out of reading through these forums was the fact that drug use in the fitness industry is not only accepted as normal; it's encouraged, glamourized, and expected.

I have to ask you this question: Do you really think those fitness models you see all over social media, on TV, and in magazines are as fit as they are because they work out and eat right? Don't fall for it! They have as much or more to gain from their bodies as do bodybuilders and women's fitness competitors, and anything more than 10 percent body fat may get them cut from the part. It's just like with the other groups I've discussed previously: When it comes to competitions based on how fit you look, steroids and other drugs will find their way into the lineup. Sometimes you may be able to tell which ones are on drugs and sometimes you will have no idea, but chances are, something with a little extra punch is floating around in their blood—something totally unnatural. What about the really unnatural looking guys walking around in gyms who aren't involved in any type of fitness competitions or modeling—are they riding the roid train too?

The Big Guys

This next group of steroid users is more entertaining for me than anything. For the most part, this group doesn't participate in contests, other than breaking records for posing in front of the mirror after every set they do. They are the big guys roaming around in every gym who are usually wearing tank tops or other shirts that are way too small, they sport that red swollen look, and they have those discolored pimple scars all over their backs, shoulders, and upper arms. And it never fails; most everyone in the gym glorifies them because they're so big. These guys definitely draw attention, and most of them are willing to give out their workout advice, but just like the bodybuilders, they're going to hold back their biggest secret of all. They don't bother me much, and like I said, they are pretty entertaining. But when they start bringing in their pharmaceutical grade "supplements" for distribution in the gym, things can get out of hand very fast. I've seen these guys have their little meetings in the parking lot or corner of the gym. The dead giveaways are their brief and subtle head nods and their hushed conversations as they constantly look around to see who's watching them. I've seen other things too that you won't believe, and this next story is definitely one I'll never forget.

Back in the early '90s when I first started my personal training business, I was unknowingly working smack dab in the middle of one of the biggest steroid rings to ever exist. I'm talking about hourly transactions of steroids and GHB, needles lying on the floor or in the commode, and vials of who knows what in trash cans and on the floor, every single day. This was a common occurrence, but there was one week that was beyond anything normal, even under these circumstances. It all started with two trainers passing out right in the middle of their clients' sessions. One guy was sitting on a box watching his client do the hack squat when all of a sudden, he just fell off the box, laid on the floor, and started snoring really loud! No kidding! The other trainer was watching his client warm up on the treadmill when he took his nose dive and went to dreamland. Both of these guys were heavy steroid users, and to make things interesting, they both were taking GHB as well. I'll get into exactly what GHB is in Chapter 4, but for now, just know it's like liquid ecstasy and was commonly referred to as the "date rape drug." I remember a very uneasy nervousness all over that gym, and I could sense that something big was coming. I wasn't disappointed. Over the next few days, at least three trainers somehow disappeared, and even their clients didn't know where they were. Several of the really big guys who worked out there disappeared as well. Then the news came: All of these guys who disappeared had been busted for distribution of a controlled substance called anabolic steroids, and the story was that the cops were working their way through to take this whole ring down. They were definitely off to a strong start.

The worst part is, one guy I knew very well disappeared too, but he wasn't arrested; he was on the bad end of a drug deal gone bad, had his jaw broken, and was in the hospital trying to recover. At that time, treatment for GHB withdrawal was nonexistent, so it was a big guess as to how to treat the symptoms. Unfortunately, this man ended up dying in that hospital from various complications; yet another casualty as the big ring came crashing down. As it turned out, there were a whole bunch of people involved in this steroid ring; I'm talking about doctors, attorneys, and very prominent business people. It all made sense to me because all of these people were the same ones walking around looking like bodybuilders but never competing. And wouldn't you know it, they all disappeared as well, really quickly. I left that gym the very next week because it was just too crazy for me, and from what I heard, things continued to get worse and more people went "missing." Steroids are bad news any way you look at it, and as you can see, there are many people taking part. If you see a man or a woman who looks unnaturally big and fit, the chances are, unnatural is exactly what they are. But what about the older population, especially the ones who are in really good shape? Could it be that they are trading in their prunes for a new and improved kind of super juice?

60 is the New 20

We've covered several different groups who use steroids and lie about it, but there's another group you might not expect that is turning sixty into the new twenty. You can see a few of them in the gym, several on TV, and even more on social media who have sixty-year-old faces but twenty-year-old bodies, and they all lie about their newfound method of age reversal. I love seeing the older folks taking part in exercise and adding years to their lives, but when I see an older man or woman walking around with the body of a well-built twenty-something, I have to laugh. Look, I'm all for chasing the fountain of youth, but please don't act like your twenty-something body came from just working out and eating right. I see these people in gyms, on social media, and all over fitness advertisements flexing their fake muscles and pushing some kind of "breakthrough supplement," telling everyone that they can look just like they do at any age. Again, it's all a big load of BS.

Some of these older folks are doing the hardcore drugs the bodybuilders are doing, but I think most of them are getting it straight from their doctors. All it takes is getting a little blood test, and if their testosterone numbers are anywhere near being low or normal for their age... presto! A testosterone prescription is handed over, the magic beans do their job, and the body magically becomes years younger. I can actually understand and even agree that there are a lot of people who can benefit from testosterone and other hormone therapies. But just because you're older and your doctor prescribed your brand-new youth serum or under-the-skin super pellet, you're not exempt from telling the truth. Enjoy your newfound youth, but be honest when people ask you where you found it. And what about the middle-aged groups—are they jumping on the testosterone-booster bandwagon even at a relatively young age? You better believe they are!

The forty-somethings are getting the exact same prescriptions from their doctors as the older folks, and when people ask them how they got into such great shape, they lie like dogs and say they started working out harder and eating better. It's easier to believe from someone in their forties, but it's still all a big fat lie. So are people younger than forty getting the big testosterone boost, or is this the bottom line as far as age goes? No way; it's not even close. I know many men in their twenties and early thirties who are getting roided up with the approval of their doctors, but there's no way they're going to admit it. And just like with all the other groups I've talked about, men aren't the only ones who are firing up their pituitary glands with steroids and growth hormones; the women want theirs stimulated too.

Oh yes, women are doing a lot more than Botox and fillers to stay young and virile; they're standing in line for their subcutaneous timed-release testosterone pellets and steroid cocktails as well. Remember when we talked about the women in fitness contests and how most of them take steroids? The only difference is most of the women who get testosterone treatments from their doctors are older and do not compete, but they're still on something. The percentage of women taking part in the big testosterone boom is growing every day, and based on what I've seen, I'd say that women are 25–35 percent of the low-testosterone market.

Overall, I think it's harmless for our aging population to use testosterone, HGH, and other hormone treatments to look and feel younger. As a matter of fact, lying about taking it for these reasons is pretty much harmless except under two conditions: First, when someone is asking for fitness advice from a person taking testosterone, and the person says that all they do is exercise and eat right. This is misleading and sets people up for a big disappointment when they follow this advice and still don't end up looking anything like the person using the hormones. Second, it is a blatant lie when a person taking testosterone is selling fitness products such as personal training, supplements, diet plans, fitness equipment, or anything else fitness related without disclosing the fact that they are taking testosterone and other drugs. This is fraud, regardless of whether or not a doctor prescribed the drugs, and just like all the other groups in this chapter, they need to be called out.

Drugs are everywhere in the fitness industry, and even though you might not see needles, out-of-control roid rages, or steroid busts, the evidence is glaring from one end to the other, leaving this industry full of a lot of things besides health.

From bodybuilders, women's physique contestants, and other fitness athletes; to fitness models, the big guys walking around the gym, and everyone taking part in the big testosterone boom; steroids and other PEDs are as common as protein drinks. Oh, they want you to believe that all they do is work out all day, eat healthy, and take vitamins, but the truth is, they have a great drug connection, and it may even be their doctor. Exercise may be in their blood, but that's not all that's in there. Maybe they're just taking testosterone to improve their overall look and to feel better; or maybe they're taking a whole concoction of muscle-building, youth-sparing, wonder drugs to keep their bodies looking like walking road maps.

> No matter what the fitness industry wants you to
> believe, the fountain of youth has not been found, but
> there's a whole lot of stuff people are taking that makes
> it look like they're swimming in it.

There's a fountain all right, and it's been around for a very long time, but it's definitely not youth that's flowing through it.

4 The Fountain of Juice

The Synthetic Shortcut

Oh yes, the juice is definitely flowing, and as you saw in the previous chapter, the fitness industry is drinking up. I'm not talking about wheat grass, carrot juice, or a blender full of someone's magical pyramid scheme drink. I'm talking about a syringe full of vitamin J, the juice of champions. You definitely won't see this kind of juice in any health food store, vitamin shop, or in the organic section of the grocery store. But you can still very easily find it at your local gym, with a quick trip to Mexico, or even at your doctor's office; just be prepared to pay the price. Since the fountain of youth refuses to be found, the fountain of juice is taking over as the quick fix to the ultimate body, and people all over the fitness industry are lining up to jump right in. And so, the fitness facade continues as people in all areas of sports and fitness are bogusly boosting their bodies with drugs as they lie to our faces about their "clean living" and "dedication to wellness."

From reading the last chapter, you know exactly who it is that's all juiced up; now let's look at exactly what they're taking. In this chapter, I'm going to walk you through the wild world of steroids, explain what each drug does, and tell you which ones are the most popular with certain groups. I'm also going to show you how these illegal drugs change hands without the buyers and sellers getting caught. And here we go again with the deceit, trickery, and fraudulent activities that go hand in hand with what's supposed to be the healthiest industry of all. The different types of steroids are astounding, but what they can do to the human body is absolutely crazy. Let's take a closer look at the a la carte menu of steroid madness and see who's ordering what.

I'm going to start with the biggest and baddest steroids around. These are the go-to roids when it comes to gaining huge amounts of muscle in a short amount of time, but beware: A few of these are well known for leading to severe and uncontrollable aggression; that's always a nice characteristic. These are also the ones that cause the penis to wilt into the little shriveled stalk that just lies around like a broken twig wishing it could. Such a great trade-off for all that new muscle. I wonder what the girlfriends and wives of these steroid users think. These are the same hardcore steroids that were extremely popular back in the Arnold days and still are today because of their super potency. As a matter of fact, it's steroids like these that keep the dialysis machines in high demand because they absolutely kill the kidneys. And that liver that's as tough as nails—it's going downhill too. Let's take a closer look at the Menu of Muscle and see exactly what poisons people are picking to get their swole on.

The Menu of Muscle – Pick Your Poison

Super-Roids – Going Old School

Dianabol: Most commonly referred to as Dbol, the granddaddy of them all. Dianabol is one of the most popular anabolic steroids of all time, and it was the second anabolic steroid ever created, right after testosterone. This steroid was developed by an American physician for the sole purpose of enhancing the athletic performance of US Olympic athletes, and it worked. Since its inception in 1958, Dianabol has been a favorite of nearly every performance enhancing athlete on earth. The number one benefit of Dianabol is growth, but an increase in strength is a close second. A person using Dbol can gain as much as twenty pounds in only a few weeks; sometimes even more. While growth is the number one reason many people use Dbol, many athletes, especially advanced performance athletes, use Dbol to break through plateaus. In most cases, Dbol is used at the beginning of a bulking cycle to kick things off. Who takes it? This steroid is very popular with bodybuilders, strength athletes, and the really big guys walking around the gym. As far as women using this steroid, it's really limited to female bodybuilders because of the huge amount of muscle that comes with using it. I've seen plenty of women who have used this drug. Have you seen these guys—I mean women? They're huge! OK, on to super roid number two.

Deca-Durabolin: Commonly referred to as Deca, Deca-Durabolin is one of the most popular anabolic steroids of all time. Without question, it's one of the best mass builders on the planet, but it's also used to help people cut up. This is another very strong steroid that is tops on the list for bodybuilders, powerlifters, and athletes requiring strength and size. And if you really want to look all puffed up, swole, and walk around with your arms all bowed out to the sides, you can take Dianabol and Deca at the same time.

Bye-bye penis, balls, and sex life, and hello back acne and marbles for nuts; more great trade-offs.

Anadrol: Also referred to as the A-bomb, Anadrol is known as the drug of choice for powerlifters and strongman contestants. This is another steroid people take to pack on muscle as fast as they can. Per all the research I did, it was determined that this particular steroid aggressively stimulates estrogen production, which is the main female hormone. And guess what? Yep, the guys who take it get what's called "bitch tits" or gynecomastia, which basically means swollen male breast tissue. Another sexy characteristic for their girlfriends and wives to enjoy. It's also a dead giveaway when you see it; it's really nasty looking and reminds me of cow udders. Other steroids typically produce this side effect as well, but this particular steroid is well known for it. This steroid also makes the user retain tons of water, so not only do they get to have swollen and protruding nipples, they get to walk around looking like a water balloon that's about to pop as well. Nope; I'll pass.

Testosterone Suspension: This form of testosterone is referred to as the Cadillac of all forms of testosterone for several reasons: It's pure testosterone with no ester, it's really fast acting, and it leaves the body very quickly, so it's harder to pick up with testing. This pure testosterone can do it all: It packs on the muscle, increases recovery times, improves stamina and endurance, and, of course, reduces body fat by raising a person's total metabolic rate. For these reasons, it's the testosterone of choice with athletes who face random drug testing because, for the most part, it's completely out of their systems and hard to detect in just twenty-four to seventy-two hours after the last injection. Think about this for a minute—an athlete in any sport can take this particular steroid all the way through their training and stop taking it three or four days before being tested, and they stand a good chance of getting away scot-free. In the next chapter, I'll show you all the ways people get around drug testing, and it's absolutely ridiculous! It's easy to see why athletes across the board would be tempted to use this steroid, and my bet is, almost all of them do it, especially professional athletes.

Winstrol: Remember the story I told you about the huge amounts of steroids being distributed in the gym where I began my personal training career? Winstrol is a name I heard constantly thrown around like it was a new kind of protein drink. Ha! I was so ignorant at that time. It's not only a popular anabolic steroid, it may also be the most well-known anabolic steroid of all time. Since its inception, Winstrol has been front and center in many high-profile steroid busts. In fact, Winstrol was part of one of the most important steroid scandals of all time when Canadian sprinter Ben Johnson tested positive for the hormone during the 1988 Summer Olympics. It was this very steroid that would lead to the US Congress classifying anabolic steroids as schedule III controlled substances through the Anabolic Steroids Control Act of 1990. Without question, the enhancement of athletic performance is one of this steroid's greatest benefits; therefore, it sits at the top of steroid wish lists for athletes at all levels. This steroid greatly increases strength, but it is not well known for producing much in the way of muscle growth, which is a dead giveaway of steroid use. Yet another attribute that makes this steroid appealing to many athletes.

So there you go—a list and description of some of the most powerful steroids flowing through the fitness industry like brand-new, hell-on-wheels, pre-workout drinks. These next few steroids are still in the biggest and baddest category, but they come with a bonus benefit. In addition to gaining huge amounts of muscle and strength, these are the steroids most known for increased aggression and uncontrollable rage. Let's see, people are taking a substance that makes them unbelievably big and strong and susceptible to episodes of uncontrollable rage. Another great idea in the world of fitness.

A Session of Aggression

Trenbolone Acetate (Finaplix): Most commonly referred to as Tren. This is one of the most popular steroids in strength sports and fitness contests for many reasons, and it's a goldmine for anyone looking to increase their power output. Information from the Association Against Steroid Abuse explained, "There are many powerful anabolic androgenic steroids at our disposal and many carry with them powerful characteristics, but if there is one steroid that stands above all the rest in terms of raw power it is without question Trenbolone."[6] The association also explained that Trenbolone was originally developed to beef up livestock.

Can you believe that? If Trenbolone can beef up livestock, just imagine what it can do to the human body. I can't tell you how many times I've heard this steroid being talked about by both men and women, and after doing my research, I now know that they are complete idiots for taking this rubbish. And to make this drug even better, it has the wonderful side effect of causing an increase in aggression. Nice! I wonder how many roid rages exploded from taking this bad boy.

Mibolerone: Here's another great idea—let's use a steroid that originated as a drug used by veterinarians to alter the ovulating cycle of female dogs to keep them from going into heat. Wow! How could this possibly end badly? In powerlifting circles, this is a well-known, pre-contest bad boy that is quite popular. It can dramatically increase your aggression in a very short amount of time. Since aggression is a key attribute in all strength sports, powerlifters seem to like this more than bodybuilders. Other sports where this steroid is taking center ring is MMA and professional boxing. Since it clears the system fast as well, it makes it popular with MMA fighters who are now under the scrutiny of rigid drug testing. It is also rumored in the boxing world that a certain fighter who was already at the top of the aggression chart would take this steroid minutes before he fought. This same boxer mistook the ear of his opponent for a hamburger in a very popular fight. Do you know who it is? Throughout my career as a personal trainer I've witnessed several close calls in the gym involving hyper-aggressive individuals. I've watched guys and gals get steaming mad when someone simply walks in front of them, asks them if they can work in on the machine they're currently using, or just looks at them the wrong way. I honestly don't see how these individuals make it outside the gym with their mean mugging and "I hate everybody" attitudes.

There are other outrageous muscle producing steroids on the market, but these are the ones that come through the needles of the really huge men and women. In terms of professional athletes and the guys walking through the doors of the local T clinics, the steroids they use may be something a little different. Now they can still up their doses or add one of the steroids we just talked about to their cycle and turn into a pissed off walking boulder, but for the most part, these steroids aren't quite in the same ball park. But just like with anything, it can get way out of hand very quickly and often it does. Let's take a look at the steroids in a class I call The Performance Package and see exactly who it is that's stepping up to the plate to get a little more pep in their step.

The Performance Package

Human Growth Hormone (HGH): The real McCoy! Human growth hormone is not a steroid; it's a protein-based peptide hormone naturally released by the pituitary and controlled by the hypothalamus. The biggest benefits of using HGH are tissue growth and repair, and body fat reduction, all of which will translate into a physique that possesses a more powerful metabolism. Although very expensive, HGH is extremely popular with professional athletes and others who can afford it. Any guess why it's so popular with athletes other than its healing and recuperative powers? It's all in the testing baby! At present, HGH can only be detected through blood testing, which is also very limiting because it can only detect HGH taken twenty-four to forty-eight hours prior to blood screening. And as far as urine testing, it won't pick up HGH one bit.

Testosterone: The big T! The most popular steroid around. Even though the human body (both male and female) produces testosterone naturally, the production naturally starts to decline once we reach twenty-five, making it harder to gain and keep lean muscle as we age. This is why testosterone is the exact steroid at the helm of every single testosterone treatment clinic going today. But for those taking testosterone outside of these clinics, it's typically just the tip of the iceberg of what they're taking. The "if some is good, then more is better" philosophy prompts most steroid users to take three or more steroids at the same time. This is referred to as stacking. Testosterone is the king and it's extremely popular across the board with steroid users, including athletes at all levels. From the research I've done, testosterone use by athletes is as common as sports drinks on the sidelines, and there's plenty to go around.

Omnadron and Sustanon-250: Both of these are types of testosterone and they were very popular steroids in the '80s and '90s, but because many labs began to counterfeit them, their popularity dropped a bit. Basically, both of these substances are a combination of four different testosterones that cover all bases, including increased muscle mass and strength, increased metabolism, increased fat-burning ability, and increased recuperation from training. These substances are ideal for testosterone replacement therapy and are used by many if not all T clinics today. Think of them as steroid cocktails, which is exactly the term I've heard many people use in the gym, including women.

Primobolan: This steroid is similar to the other testosterones I've mentioned so far but it isn't as potent. It also doesn't cause bitch tits, and it is considered a better fat burner than all other testosterones combined. Overall, it's not a very popular steroid because it takes a lot of it to see any change, and it's expensive. Even the shortcut isn't short enough for some cheaters.

Testosterone Enanthate: Many consider this to be the most popular testosterone there is simply because it's very available, affordable, and it works really well. Many articles I've read stated that this type of testosterone is easily tolerated by both men and women. Oh yes, women are all over testosterone, and if you watch real closely, you'll see it walking around in the gym or on TV. And those fitness instructors... watch out; the look they're sporting may be from a syringe full of magic juice instead of their claims of nonstop exercise and strict diets.

Anavar: I call this the gender friendly steroid because both men and women can tolerate this steroid fairly well. In fact, this is the single most female friendly anabolic steroid on the market. This tends to make many men assume the steroid won't be strong enough for them, and while it's not a strong mass promoting steroid, it can be extremely beneficial to the male athlete. As a bonus, some studies have shown Anavar also has the ability to greatly improve and maximize cardio-vascular endurance. I can't see why this would benefit athletes, can you? Without question, Anavar is one of the best-known steroids for the enhancement of athletic performance. This steroid will boost strength significantly; it may not do so as robustly as some steroids, but the change will be notable. By taking this drug, athletes can gain strength and endurance without large buildups in muscle mass. You can easily see why this is a gem within the athletic community.

Before I move on, I want to make a strong point here. Steroid use is rampant in every nook and cranny of the fitness industry, and as you can see, it's not limited to professional sports. I am constantly warning parents who have kids involved in sports to be very aware of the images and ideas to which their children are exposed. These kids see the big guys in the gym, on TV, and on their teams as well, and they can't help but be envious of their muscled-up bodies and athletic ability. But there's another threat of which all parents need to be aware.

> If you're a parent and you're hiring a trainer, coach, or bodybuilder to take your kid through workouts, pay very close attention to what goes on inside that gym.

Just the other day when I was working out, I saw three trainers in a group having one of those secretive conversations. I could have guessed what was being talked about, but I wanted to see for sure, so I got kind of close to where they were and turned my music off. I still had my headphones in so they thought I was listening to my music. Sure enough, these idiots were discussing how much

Deca-Durabolin and Clenbuterol they were taking, and how they were told by some other muscle head how to add three or four other steroids to their stacks. One trainer even listed five or six different steroids he was taking to get ready for his big show. One of the trainers was new to everything because the other two were teaching this guy what to take and when to take it. And the craziest part? They were also telling him what to take to avoid all the water gain he's about to get. It was absolutely crazy that I was hearing this conversation as I was writing this very chapter. What happened next is the very reason I warn all parents about who trains and coaches their kids. As they were talking, one of them said, "Hey, be quiet, be quiet; here comes my next client." And the client he was referring to was a kid. The kid looked to be around fourteen or fifteen years old, and he walked up right in the middle of these roid heads, and after a little talk and a couple of handshakes, the kid and his trainer walked off and began their workout.

Remember, steroids are very easy to get, and the information on exactly which ones to buy and how to take them is everywhere. This is some pretty crazy stuff, right? Buying steroids is as easy as walking into a restaurant, looking at a menu, and placing your order. I'll take the Deca special with a side order of Anabol and testosterone, and could you please put the Winstrol on the side? As funny as this sounds, this is exactly how it goes down when someone places their order at their local "all-you-can-inject buffet." And I can hear the dealer now… "Sorry, we're all out of Deca, but I can substitute some Trenbolone for you with a fifty-dollar up-charge."

The world of steroids is indeed crazy a**, and to add to the craziness, most users take even more drugs to hide the really unnatural side effects from using steroids. You know, things like males growing female breast tissue, ruining their kidneys and livers, and turning their bodies into walking water supplies. Take a look at this list I call Hide and Sneak, where you can see the drugs of choice for the big roid cover up; it's all the rage!

Hide and Sneak

Clomid, Arimidex, Aromasin: These drugs have become popular in many performance enhancing circles as drugs to combat issues of estrogen buildup, which will more than likely lead to gynecomastia (bitch-tit syndrome). These drugs also have a role in post-steroid-cycle therapy to increase and stimulate natural testosterone production after a person gets off the roids. Basically, these drugs counteract the effects of the other drugs by reducing the newly developed female breast tissue and re-inflating the balls. So really, it's an exchange of breasts for balls. Wow! Glad it's their balls and not mine.

Lasix, Aldactone, Dyazide: These drugs are all diuretics used by physique athletes such as bodybuilders and women's fitness pageant contestants, and are also common within the modeling communities. These drugs will give athletes tighter and drier physiques, making them look extremely lean and hard. As far as performance athletes in professional sports and especially boxing, MMA, and wrestling, these athletes might use these drugs to help them meet a specific weight class. One huge problem with these drugs is dehydration. It not only gets rid of water in the body, it also depletes the body of sodium and other electrolytes. Use of these diuretics is very common throughout the fitness industry; just another smart decision made by the industry that cares. Right! And by the way, diuretics are banned in professional sports because they mask the use of steroids. Imagine that!

Nolvadex: Anytime synthetic testosterone or other steroids are put into the body, a person's natural testosterone production greatly diminishes or stops altogether. Nolvadex is the drug of choice to rekindle natural testosterone production after a person cycles off steroid use, and boy is it in high demand. With every article I read on steroid use, this drug was mentioned as a post-cycle must. I've heard stories of severe depression from steroid users who cycled off steroids and didn't do anything to restore their natural testosterone production. And whose fault is this? It's almost like booking a one-way flight and then getting mad and depressed because you have no way to get home. Let's see, I'm going to take a drug that will give me a whole lot more of what my body already makes to the point where I actually stop making it myself. And then I'm going to stop taking the first drug and take a different drug to help my body start making the first drug again. Sounds rational and smart to me; how about you?

This whole book is about lies, and steroids fit right in. But the lies definitely don't stop here. There's another group of drugs that falsify fitness and really bring out the fake abs. Just pop a few of these fat fryers, do a little cardio, and bam! Instant six-pack! But, of course, that newfound leanness is from a perfect workout and eating plan, right? As common as I knew drug use to be in the fitness industry, I was shocked at the unbelievable number of people from all walks of life who support the lipid lies and claim their instant and miraculous fat burning to be from their "extra effort." This next group of drugs have one job: to burn fat. And they do not let their users down. Take a look at the drugs that fall under my list of Fat Losers, and the big fat lie will become very clear.

Fat Losers

Clenbuterol (Clen): This incredibly popular drug is a stimulant and is not a steroid, but it is well known for having anabolic qualities. It was first used to treat asthma and other related breathing disorders, but a lot has changed. This is a very popular fat burner for many people, including anabolic steroid users, competitive bodybuilders, all fitness competitors, and athletes. But what makes it so common is that numerous non-competitors and non-steroid users, including many actors and actresses, use and enjoy this drug as a fat burner just as much as anyone else.

The article, "Clenbuterol: The Most Popular Hollywood Secret," on *newcolonist.com* explained that, while Hollywood's attractive stars might swear that their stick-thin bodies are the result of clean eating and exercise, "The current buzz in Hollywood is that Clenbuterol can help you lose weight, get in shape for a red-carpet event, and even get you that exclusive size-zero body that you crave."[7]

Believe me, there's a lot more going on in Hollywood than eating right and exercise, and Clenbuterol is only one of several things these famous folks take to look fit. From my research, I also found that many male and female models, professional cheerleaders, and others who rely on their aesthetic look to make a living are the biggest users of this drug. Another fact I found was that Clenbuterol was extremely popular with people who just work out and want to be leaner. Here's something to note: Although approved in most countries, Clenbuterol has never been approved by the US Food and Drug Administration (FDA). Clenbuterol has a unique legal loophole making it illegal to sell but legal to use and possess, and it's not on the controlled substance list. So how does it work? Simply put, Clenbuterol increases the body's core temperature and, in turn, increases the individual's metabolism of triglycerides and body fat. Clenbuterol is an extremely simple compound but highly effective, and it's in every gym in the world.

Albuterol: This drug is very similar to Clenbuterol and has been labeled as the super ephedrine. Both are fat burners, but one big difference is that albuterol only lasts for about four to six hours whereas Clenbuterol lasts up to thirty-six hours. Basically, people who take albuterol have to take two to three times as much to match the fat-burning pace of Clenbuterol.

Ephedrine: You remember this one, don't you? Yes, it's illegal to sell but just like all of the other drugs we've talked about, you can find it if you look around. And just like steroids, it's legal in several other countries. Just like with the other fat-burning drugs, ephedrine speeds up metabolism, burns body fat at a higher rate, and suppresses the appetite.

Ephedrine was by far the most popular fat-burning drug used until it was declared illegal to sell in 2004.

Cytomel: Here's an interesting one. Cytomel is a thyroid hormone that increases the level of adenosine triphosphate (ATP) in the body. This means that the body will have more energy both during everyday activities and especially during workouts. The increase in ATP means the increase in the level of metabolism, which means more energy for the body from fat reserves. Yep, just another drug-induced fat burn concealed by cardio lies.

There are several other fat-burning drugs, but these are the most commonly used in the fitness industry, both in and out of competitions. In case I haven't mentioned this, fat-burning drugs are almost always associated with steroid use. You see, it's just not enough to pack on all that lean muscle, they have to take other drugs to help burn the fat away so everyone can see just how big and lean they are. It's a crazy cycle within a cycle, and the lengths to which some people go to look fit is absolutely amazing to me. Here's another drug I want to show you, which really blew me away when it showed up in my research. It made absolutely no sense to me because I couldn't bridge the gaps with how this drug would work, but now I see. You're not going to believe this, but insulin is commonly used by many bodybuilders, athletes, and others trying to add mounds of muscle. Yep, insulin!

Insulin: Of all the powerful anabolic hormones available, very few are as powerful as insulin. Absolutely shocking to me! Without question, competitive bodybuilders are the number one users of this hormone (with the exception of diabetics who need it), with athletes coming in a strong second. When people who are not diabetic inject insulin, their bodies are able to process larger amounts of food beyond what they normally eat, particularly proteins and carbohydrates. They are able to absorb their protein at a higher degree, and they are able to maximize the benefit of each and every gram of carbohydrates they consume. With this amazing ability to process nutrition at a much higher than normal rate, the body also starts to increase natural growth factors, which triggers an overall increase in body mass. You can see why bodybuilders and athletes would want to include this in their drug arsenal. Now here's the kicker: If someone is injecting insulin, for non-diabetic reasons of course, it's an almost 100 percent guarantee they are using steroids as well. If they didn't use steroids with their abnormally high levels of insulin, they would get fat, plain and simple. And, of course, they can always add a few of the fat-burning drugs we just talked about to fix that problem too. What about buffing up the blood—are there methods other than using steroids and fat burners that the glorified cheaters use? You bet there are!

Can you see the pattern here? It's like it's never enough. As if steroids and fat-burning drugs didn't tax their organs enough, these users poke yet more holes in their bodies and inject other drugs or chemicals to get just a little more advantage. But it's OK that their livers and kidneys are thirty years older than they should be; they'll just take other drugs to fix those too. Remember, it's all for health. Why do I keep thinking of a particular dwarf? Let's dig a little deeper into what these Dope Heads are doing and see how desperate they really are for the glory.

Dope Heads

Blood Doping: This even sounds horrible to me, but it's just another way a lot of people attain their fake fitness. So what the heck is it anyway? Blood doping is simply artificially boosting the blood's ability to bring more oxygen to working muscles. There's one sport which immediately comes to mind when I think of blood doping—professional cycling. Remember the gentleman named Lance Armstrong and the huge steroid controversy that hung over him like a cheap, wet suit? There you go! Blood doping is a big problem in all sports, and there are three main ways it's done.

1. *Blood Transfusions* – I know, pretty crazy, right? They do this in one of two ways: They either get a transfusion of their own blood, which they had taken and stored in the past, or they get a transfusion from another person. This fresh blood is full of oxygen and tons of red blood cells and not depleted like the blood currently in their body because of extreme training and grueling events.

2. *Erythropoietin (EPO) Injections* – EPO is a hormone that is naturally secreted from the kidneys, but, of course, natural just won't cut it for many people. This is another absurd method to get an athletic edge. Injecting EPO will force the kidneys to produce more than normal red blood cells, which means more oxygen. This leads to greater athletic endurance and performance. This is a very popular means of blood doping; it came up on every piece of research I viewed, and the world of professional cycling was cited as a main user.

3. *Synthetic Oxygen Carriers* – These are chemicals that have the ability to carry oxygen. There are two types: HBOCs (hemoglobin-based oxygen carriers) and PFCs (perfluorocarbons). I had never heard of these (as I'm sure you haven't either) but they're worth noting. Injecting chemicals into the body—yeah, that's healthy.

That's a heck of a lot of drug use, isn't it? And every one of these is illegal to use without a prescription. But, as you can see, that really doesn't stop anyone. These drugs are everywhere, and most of the fitness industry is pumped full of them.

What about the other drugs—you know, the ones that used to be available at every supplement store in the United States that were once legal and are now in the same class as steroids? And the ones that, according to some people, "aren't really steroids," like prohormones and SARMs (selective androgen receptor modulators)? No matter what your beast-mode friend told you, bro, these are steroids, and most of them are illegal. Let's look at prohormones and SARMs a little closer to see exactly why they're referred to as The Other Steroids.

The Other Steroids

Prohormones: Prohormones are not technically hormones. Instead, they are unique chemical compounds that increase the effects of existing hormones within the body. Basically, prohormones are a weaker form of anabolic steroids, and don't let anyone convince you otherwise. And they work; maybe not nearly as fast or as well as the other steroids we talked about in this chapter, but they do unnaturally alter the human body and its ability to perform. On December 18, 2014, President Obama signed DASCA, the Designer Anabolic Steroid Control Act of 2014, which banned the use and sale of most prohormones. And the prohormones that are still legal—they are merely watered-down versions, and they do not contain the same testosterone precursors as the original prohormones. Either way, it's still an unnatural thing to take to achieve greater athletic performance and/or a bigger, leaner body. The whole thing is shady, and it doesn't really matter to me if someone takes them or not, until they lie about using them. And since the feds put their foot down on the sale and use of prohormones, the relentlessly increasing demand in the fitness industry for another shortcut to a better body led to yet another drug to fill the void of banned prohormones. And just like that, SARMs were delivered as the new go-to drugs.

SARMs: These are nonsteroidal compounds that still activate the androgen receptors, and according to my research, using them typically gives similar results to a prohormone or light steroid cycle. These drugs took center stage in 2014 and 2015 when prohormones became illegal, but at the same time, SARMs are illegal to sell and are just another drug that resides on the banned substance list of every professional sport out there. I'm not going to go into the different SARMs and their descriptions because they all pretty much have the same effect: They unnaturally increase the ability of the human body to gain lean muscle and increase athletic performance, just like all the other drugs I've discussed in this chapter. And as far as the challenges of finding these drugs, they might as well just put them in vending machines. There's one more drug I want to show you that was very popular among bodybuilders back in the '90s and early 2000s, and from what I've heard, it's still in heavy circulation. I'm talking about gamma-hydroxybutyrate (GHB), more commonly known as the date rape drug.

GHB: At one time, this drug was sold over the counter at supplement and health food stores, just like prohormones were. And when people started dying from taking it, they thought it was best to take it down, but this didn't stop anyone. People were making this stuff in their garages and storage sheds by the gallons and turning huge profits. Bodybuilders and other fitness fanatics would swear that it had anabolic qualities and would make them bigger and leaner. Remember those trainers I told you about who passed out right in the middle of their sessions? Yep, they were on GHB. I remember exactly how they would take it too. They called it "a cap of G" because they would carry it around in a plain water bottle, and when they wanted a snort they would pour it into the water bottle cap and drink it, right there on the gym floor. And even though many people overdosed on it (and several died), it was commonly passed around in gyms just like steroids and other drugs. Is it around today? Oh, I'm sure it is, and the lies and stupidity are right there with it.

The lists of different drugs go on and on with no end in sight, and if someone wants to take them, they'll find them as easy as they find their morning coffee. The sources of these drugs are a heck of a lot closer than you may think, and believe me, the dealers are dealing. So exactly how do people get their hands on all of these drugs? Are they going out of the country and hoping the drug dogs don't blow up on them when they try to sneak them back in, or do they leave that stuff to the dealers and just meet in parking lots and trade their money for their new muscle in a bottle? Finding steroids is almost like finding fish; you can try to catch them yourself, or you can simply walk into any grocery store or restaurant and have them brought right to you ready to go. There are several ways people go about finding their roids of choice, and I have listed them here in my list of Synthetic Sources.

Synthetic Sources

The Gym

Now, this is a great fishing hole! The big fish are there, and if someone plays their cards right, this can be their one-stop shop for every drug they could ever need. In the very gym where I started my personal training career, you didn't even have to ask; people walked up and asked you if there was anything you needed. No kidding! Remember those quiet little meetings I mentioned that go on over by the squat rack or in another corner of the gym? Chances are, that's exactly what's going on, or it's well on its way. There's no mistaking who it is that's got the connection; it's just a matter of getting closer to the group. In my opinion, the gym is the ultimate steroid buying hot spot simply because of all I've seen over nearly three decades in the fitness business.

Those gym bags the big guys are carrying around have
a lot more than weight belts and Creatine in them;
there's also a flashing sign that says Pharmacy Open!

Online Steroid Forums

During my research I found several of these forums and let me tell you, I felt like I needed a shower after reading what these guys were discussing. It's 100 percent steroids in these forums, and you can tell who's in the clique and who's not. You can also read between the lines and see the deals going down right there on the screen. There is even steroid forum etiquette where they tell you to not come right out and ask where you can get steroids. "Steroid Etiquette"... hmm. But in any case, this is a popular place where many people slide their way into steroid circles and get their synthetic substances in an off-line manner.

Buying Online

I've heard countless people talking about online steroid shops and how they get anything they want through a website, and they swear by the quality of their online roids.

In the *WebMD* article, "Anabolic Steroid Seekers Find Easy Access," author Todd Zwillich wrote, "A simple Google search for the term 'buy anabolic steroids' yields more than 2.8 million hits. There's no way of knowing how many of the sites offer anabolic steroids as opposed to related precursors or simple placebo scams. But the sites reflect what some officials and experts say is a huge international market that promises a ready supply to almost anyone who seeks the drugs."[8]

Although I believe there are plenty of online sources where anyone can buy anabolic steroids, I also believe there are many sites selling fake steroids. As I stated before, if someone wants steroids and other illegal fitness drugs bad enough, they are sure to find them in one place or another. And if they can't find a drug connection in the local gym or online, they can take a little trip and try their luck on foreign soils.

Outside of the United States

I'm not sure how many actually do this, but buying steroids and other fitness drugs outside of the United States seems to be a go-to plan for many suppliers. I'm not sure of the validity of what one steroid user told me, but he said that one way people get steroids from other countries is to go to that country, buy the steroids, and then ship them to a post office box back in the United States. Again, I'm not sure this is accurate but it's certainly interesting. Topping the list of where people go to buy their steroids outside of the United States is Mexico. From what I have read, most of the steroids bought in

Mexico are from veterinarians and small pharmacies. And after buying them, customers either mail them back to the United States or they hold their breath and try to drive them back across the border. I'm sure you've seen the movies where the US authorities ask the car to pull to the side so they can check it. A great example of this is in the movie *Dallas Buyer's Club* when the main character, played by Matthew McConaughey, who was dressed up as a priest, was interrogated about the huge quantity of drugs he was bringing back to the United States. Great movie by the way! But I think the outcome would be quite a bit different from what happened in this movie if someone were caught with steroids coming from Mexico. There are other countries where steroids can be purchased without a prescription as well: the Bahamas, Columbia, Costa Rica, Greece, Hong Kong, India, Korea, Puerto Rico, and Thailand. I'm not sure how many people actually go this route, but I'm sure there are plenty who do.

Legal Prescriptions

Remember the section in Chapter 3, 60 is the New 20, where I talked about the big testosterone boom? Guys and gals are lining up at doctor's offices and low-T clinics all over the country to get their testosterone topped off. Yep, this is a legal place to both buy and use steroids. Even though this is the legal way to get it done, people are still hiding behind it as they lie about their newfound fitness. Enough said.

There you go—the dubious drug roundup that's alive and well within our fitness industry. The funny thing is, I didn't even come close to listing all the drugs available, and I'm sure there are other ways of getting drugs I didn't list, but I think you get my point. I know I covered some of this previously when describing what each drug does, but I want to cap off this chapter with one more list. My dad used to always tell me that most things aren't what they seem to be, and many of the people you'll get to know in life who look and act like they have it all together are often the ones who are the most lost. Boy, was he right, especially when it comes to all the steroid phonies presenting themselves as the mighty muscle ambassadors of health. In my opinion, the fitness industry is overflowing with these phonies, and their physiques are as fake as they are. But in the end, they're really cheating themselves, and I hope after reading this list and this book, you'll see exactly why. My list, After the Muscle, will give you an idea of exactly where these drug users are headed and how their bodies will follow.

After the Muscle

From Muscle to Mush

Oh yes, it's coming in a big way. Once a person stops using steroids—and they will because their organs and their over-taxed heart and arteries will make them stop—all of that lean, hard muscle they got from their wonder drugs will quickly turn into a fat, mushy mess. That's right, their insta-muscles will leave as fast as they came, leaving behind a body covered in soft fat and stretch marks. And no amount of cardio, squats, and barbell curls will get rid of it. And all of those confidence-building comments they got about their amazing bodies? Those are going to hell in a hay basket as well.

The Confidence Killer

Once the juice stops flowing and their muscles practically blow away, steroid and other drug users will be asked over and over again several confidence-destroying questions by most people they see, especially the ones at the gym: "What happened? Have you been sick?" "Wow, you've lost weight. Have you missed your workouts?" "Is everything OK? You look like you've lost a lot of weight." These are not good things to hear for anyone who works hard to maintain a healthy and strong physique, but for a person who is used to hearing praise from everyone about how big, fit, and strong they look, it kills their confidence in a heartbeat. And since steroids and other drugs play spin the bottle with a person's hormones, there's also a high likelihood of depression once they stop using. Yep, and as their emotional roller coaster drops, flips, turns, and runs out of control, they get banged around in many other ways as well.

Internal Combustion

That's right, things are heating up on the inside, and this person's not going to like what's cooking. Regardless if it was a hardcore steroid, a fat-burning drug, prohormones, or diuretics, the user's liver, kidneys, heart, and other organs take a relentless beating from the very first day of use. Oh, there are things they can take like liver detoxifiers and other "organ shielding" drugs, but there's no way around it; the organs are cooking and they'll never be the same. The exception to this is that most, if not all, doctors who prescribe testosterone treatments require periodic blood testing from their patients to ensure hormone balance, organ health, and good blood work. But beyond this, the chances of organ and natural hormone production damage are highly likely with many steroid users. But the damage doesn't stop there. There's another pill to swallow once they stop using their wonder drugs. The fast track to muscle mountain takes a bad turn, and their once fluid and painless joints start to feel like someone beat them with a hammer.

The Juiced Joint is Popping

As these users bench, squat, and curl their way through unbelievable increases in strength, their joints are dying. Is this from bad form too? Absolutely! But when your muscles are able to lift way more weight than what your joints were intended to be able to support, the rubber bands will break and cartilage will be crushed. It's like trying to pull a car out of a ditch with a jump rope; there's way too much car and way too little rope, so the rope breaks. I see guys and gals every day in the gym walking around with braces on every joint, but that's OK; they're really big and strong so they must be doing things right. And as far as their pain, I'm sure their dealer can hook them up with a dose of something that'll fix them right up.

From one end of fitness to the other, the juice bar is open and the drinks are flowing. From hardcore steroids, to fat-burning drugs, to prohormones and blood doping, shortcuts to fake fitness affect people from all walks of life, and they all lie about their lean and fit bodies. Some people say, "Let them do their drugs; they're only hurting themselves." But there are many other casualties besides shriveled-up livers, balls, and kidneys.

Users don't just do the drugs; they pass off their "superior fitness results" as being earned from nothing other than endless weight training, marathon cardio sessions, and chicken and broccoli diets, all while they pass needles and pills like they were salt and pepper.

With the fitness industry, the unnatural has become the natural. And the very industry built on real health and longevity has sold out to syringes full of shortcuts and synthetic successes.

Whichever way you choose to look at it, it's all one big fake, and the frauds need to be exposed. At first glance, the solution seems to be to establish drug testing across the entire industry, but testing the blood and urine of millions of people would be a lot more trouble than it's worth, and the results would be anything but the truth.

5 'Urine' Trouble...Unless You Know How to Cheat!

How funny would it be if gyms had steroid detectors at the front doors, and when steroids were detected in a gym member or employee, which would be all day long, a siren would go off and the name of the person and the types of drugs they were taking would be announced on the speakers? And, of course, personal trainers and group exercise instructors wouldn't be exempt; they'd have to walk through the steroid scanner too. Now that's what I call entertainment! Can you hear it? "Roid alert! Roid alert! John Doe just walked in and he's juiced to the gills with Deca, testosterone, and Winstrol, and it's all topped off with a huge dose of Clenbuterol." I would love to see the faces of those who were exposed and watch them turn twenty shades of red or get mad and run out. Why stop at gyms? We could have these steroid detectors in airports, grocery stores, restaurants, doctor's offices, and even at sporting events. Now that would be something. Can you imagine seeing someone's face on a huge screen at a sporting event and underneath would be the type of steroids they're taking? And the same would go for the players too; if steroids were detected, the player's face would be on the big screen along with their roid regimen as they're running onto the field or court. Ha! Excellence! I'd buy a ticket to see that.

Now, where roid detectors would really get interesting is at bodybuilding shows and women's fitness events. Yep, we're going to need a bigger screen to list everything they're taking. Maybe there could even be an award for most drugs in the body. They could call it the Golden Needle Award. That would be funny, but it would be even funnier at more obscure sporting events like tennis, volleyball, curling, and even bowling. Can you imagine a bowler walking up to the lane with an alarm going off and the score display flashing a list of steroids? How many shocked faces do you think there would be? And perhaps the biggest entertainment of all would be all of the fitness advertisements on social media and TV. Can you picture an infomercial showing a hot new exercise program and above each exerciser's head is a display listing the drugs they take with an arrow pointing right at them? And for the show stopper, the fitness personality who's endorsing and pushing this new exercise program would have a list of drugs they're taking flash across the screen as well. Do you think their sales would fall off a bit?

Although I know this kind of detection will never happen, it makes me laugh to think about it— especially thinking about the reactions of those who would get exposed. Shock and awe, baby!

> The truth is, testing for steroids and other illegal drugs is limited for several reasons, and with the many ways people have of masking their drug use and passing these tests, steroid testing is rapidly becoming obsolete, if it isn't already there.

The Association Against Steroid Abuse had this to say on their website: "Make no mistake; many people beat these little tests every single day. In the United States alone it is estimated at minimum 6 million adults use anabolic steroids every year. While many of these individuals are not athletes many are and the steroid testing they are put under is nothing short of a joke. To be blunt, if you possess a functioning brain and you desire to use performance enhancing drugs and you know you will be tested you can beat the test almost every time."[9]

In this chapter, I'm going to show you the different ways of testing for steroids, how often different sports teams and other athletic events test their players and participants, and last but not least, the incredible and absolutely crazy methods athletes and other people use to fake these tests. And I mean crazy! With professional sports, fitness sports, bodybuilding, and women's fitness contests, it's not a matter of who's really on steroids, it's a matter of who's truly getting tested and who's cheating the tests. With the rest of the fitness industry, they can take all the roids they want and keep lying to everyone about doing it.

So what's the protocol professional sports teams and other fitness events use to test for these champion cheaters? Do they just hand the player or participant a cup and say, "Fill 'er up," or do they try to get the truth from their veins? At this point, there are only a few tests to see who's juicing their way up the roid highway. If an athlete passes, they'll be told they're good to go. But if they fail, they'll hear three ugly words: urine trouble buddy!

So exactly who is it that throws the red flag at these cheaters and tells them to take their balls and go home? There are a few international and national agencies dedicated to managing steroid testing, its procedures, and its outcomes to determine foul play with PEDs. The main purpose of these organizations is to strike out steroids within professional sports and the Olympics, and let me tell you, they have their hands full; I just hope they know what they're really up against. Take a look so you can see exactly what role each organization has in ripping roids a new one.

Striking Out Steroids

World Anti-Doping Agency (WADA) is an international multi-sport organization that was set up by the International Olympic Committee in 1999 to stop the rise of performance enhancing drug use. This international organization set the code and standard for testing procedures and test analysis, all while constructing the official list of banned PEDs. I guess you could say they're like the Supreme Court of anti-doping agencies. All other anti-doping agencies refer to WADA for policy and procedure on testing athletes for drugs. The agency's key activities include scientific research, education, development of anti-doping capacities, and monitoring of the World Anti-Doping Code. Although there are countless labs that will analyze a steroid test, WADA has their own labs, which most professional sports teams use. And as you'll see later in this chapter, just because an organization says it follows WADA policies for their drug testing doesn't mean they enforce it.

The US Anti-Doping Agency (USADA) is the national anti-doping organization in the United States. This organization manages the anti-doping program, which includes in-competition and out-of-competition testing and processing of the test results. USADA also provides drug reference resources and athlete education for the US Olympic Committee and recognized national governing bodies of sports, their athletes, and events.

Independent Laboratories: There are countless independent labs that offer to test and analyze urine, blood, and hair follicle samples for steroids and other PEDs. Per my research, they all promise state-of-the-art test analysis, but as far as reliability and error-free results, I could not find many reviews for these companies.

Where there's competition, there are steroids and other PEDs; it's just a matter of who does and doesn't get caught. It seems these big anti-doping agencies agree with me; there's a whole lot of steroid use in this world, and somebody needs to stop it. Remember, this book is not about people taking drugs; it's about people lying about using drugs at the expense of others—big difference. It's obvious most steroid testing pertains to professional sports, with a little bit of it being done in a few fitness sports, but other than that, steroid testing in other areas of the fitness industry is unheard of. I'll be breaking down how most sports and fitness events test their athletes or competitors later in this chapter, but for now, let's look at which methods of testing are being used today and exactly what they're looking for.

Signs of a Cheater

There are three tests for steroids: urine, blood, and hair follicle, with urine tests being the most widely used. As far as what the tests are looking for, there are several indicators, but I'm going to narrow it down a bit. Basically, they are looking for performance enhancing steroids; growth factors and hormones; and masking agents like diuretics, narcotics, beta-blockers, and stimulants. The chemistry here can get way out of hand, so I'm going to keep this pretty simple and straightforward. It all starts with the big T.

Unnaturally High Levels of Testosterone

This is the first dead giveaway of steroid use. Normal blood levels of testosterone for the human male vary between 300 and 1,000 nanograms per deciliter of blood. The testosterone level for an average adult female is between 15 and 70 nanograms per deciliter of blood. So if a male athlete is tested and has a testosterone reading of over 1,200, this would be a red flag and further testing would be performed. If a female tested over 80, they would be subject to further testing as well. I've had several men tell me they went to a low testosterone clinic and their natural testosterone was tested at 400, the exact place it should be for their age. But per their "low-T doctor's advice," they should be closer to 800–1,000, which is at least double that individual's natural level. Yeah, that sounds healthy.

Testosterone/Epitestosterone Ratio

The first urine test typically performed is a testosterone/epitestosterone ratio screening test, during which a urine sample is chemically analyzed to find the ratio of the concentrations of the two hormones. The normal ratio of these two hormones is one-to-one, and WADA sets the test limit at four-to-one. If an athlete's urine sample contains more than four times as much testosterone as epitestosterone, the sample is marked as a failed test, and even if the ratio is three-to-one, further testing could be requested. If a player fails this test, they will move on to a confirmation test called an isotope ratio test.

Isotope Ratio Test

Without getting out our beakers and chemistry lab glasses, this test looks for a ratio of two carbon atoms: carbon-12 and carbon-13. Here's the skinny: Carbon-12 atoms are natural in the human body, whereas carbon-13 atoms are from synthetic sources like synthetic testosterone. If the test shows more than normal carbon-13 atoms, the athlete is a steroid cheater, plain and simple, and they will be reported. Can you imagine walking up to someone you think is taking steroids and asking, "Hey, how's your carbon-13 level?" I'm probably going to have to do it just to see their response.

HGH (Human Growth Hormone) Test

Testing for HGH is a tough task for several reasons: First, it is in and out of the body within twenty-four to forty-eight hours after injection, so the test would have to be administered on the exact day HGH was injected. Second, a blood test is really the only way to test for HGH and it's a lot more expensive than a urine test. I've read several articles stating that a urine test for HGH will be available any day now but that was as far as it went. And last, the level of HGH in the human body varies a lot from one person to the next, and it also varies in an individual throughout the day. To detect it, one would have to take several different blood tests throughout the day for several days to have a chance at detecting increased HGH levels. Because of the difficulties in testing for HGH, you can see why this hormone is high on the want list of athletes and competitors across the board.

Diuretics Testing

Diuretics are used by athletes, bodybuilders, and other fitness event contestants for two main reasons: First, diuretics increase urination, which in turn rids the body of excess water weight and sodium. Second, diuretics also remove other chemicals from the body's tissues, muscles, and blood. By chemicals, I mean chemicals related to drug use and their by-products. It's obvious why athletes and others in the fitness industry use diuretics; they're trying to cut weight, and they're trying to cheat the test. I can tell you that with every single one of the articles I read on steroids, diuretics were discussed as an essential tool needed to pass a drug test.

Narcotics Testing

A simple urinalysis or saliva test will detect narcotics even several days after use. Why test for narcotics in athletes? It's simple. Athletes can use narcotics to speed up their adrenal glands and get hyper-boosted energy to mask pain, among other unnatural uses. I'll talk about this later on, but Attention Deficit Hyperactivity Disorder (ADHD) medication is often used by pro athletes. Do they truly need the drug because of a disorder, or is it used for something else?

Beta-Blockers

Yep, some athletes even resort to taking blood pressure medication to get a performance edge. Beta-blockers are a class of medications prescribed to block the effects of adrenaline, which is a hormone produced by the adrenal glands that speeds up the heart and other functions of the body. These drugs help the heart work more efficiently by reducing blood pressure, heart rate, muscle tremors, and even anxiety. Beta-blockers also have a relaxing effect on muscle function, which as you can imagine will give every kind of athlete both a physical and mental edge. Think about archery for a minute; can you see how the calming effects of taking a beta-blocker would benefit them? The two most popular beta-blockers for athletes are propranolol and atenolol. And then there's speed.

Stimulants

This is yet another drug detected through urinalysis. This is pretty straightforward—stimulants boost energy and therefore boost performance. Athletes and everyone else can go longer and harder without fatigue when they use stimulants such as caffeine, cocaine, amphetamines, ephedrine, and even methamphetamines.

There you have it—the very things WADA, USADA, and other PED testing companies are looking for when they're testing for cheaters. There are other substances they look for as well, but for the purpose of this book, these are the big ones. As you can see, the opportunity to cheat is indeed available to everyone, athlete or not. It's always front and center in the news when a professional or Olympic athlete gets caught, but what about other sports? What about all of those other fitness sports we've talked about to this point—are they testing for steroids? And if they are, is it legitimate testing or a big joke? In my opinion, testing bodybuilders, physique contestants, and athletes for drugs is like testing the ocean for fish; they will always be there, so why waste time testing? Let's start at the top of the drug mountain and work our way down, but try not to laugh because things are about to get really funny.

'F' for Effort

BodyBuilding/Physique Contests

Because bodybuilding and other physique contests overlap in many ways and because most of them take place together, I'm going to put them in the same group; they're basically all tested in the same ways. Look, drug testing in these contests is a joke, and there's no better way to say it. Even though many of these contests say they test these guys and gals, I did my research and read through the testing policies of all of these different bodybuilding and physique leagues or federations, and my original opinion was supported. Yep, testing is practically nonexistent, and in the contests where they do test, it's nothing but a big joke!

While many of these bodybuilding contests claim they test their contestants, it's BS. Believe me, they wouldn't be able to have a contest if they tested everyone. As a matter of fact, several of these contests say absolutely nothing about drug testing because they want the biggest and freakiest bodies they can get to draw more interest to their events. As for the "all-natural" and "drug-free" events that promise stringent drug testing, their protocol for testing looks like Swiss cheese with holes so big their contestants can slide right through. Believe me, these contestants aren't worried about failing a drug test. It's almost like taking a test in school where the teacher allows everyone to bring a cheat sheet. Oh, the teacher is teaching all right, but they're also saying it's OK to cheat and even encouraging it. It's all just another example of cheating upon cheating within the fitness industry, with fraud taking center stage. Take a look at how contestants in these events are "tested," and you'll see very quickly how shady these testing procedures really are.

The Lie Protector

These are the exact testing protocols used with bodybuilding and all other physique contests, but don't expect much; the margin for error is a five-lane highway.

Steroid Free-For-All: As you might expect, several of these contests are steroid free-for-alls with absolutely no testing done. As I said in Chapter 3, it's more about who has the best chemist than who has the best workout and diet.

Drug Test for the Winners Only: This test will be given only after the contest with no other testing done before the event. So basically, a contestant can take all the drugs they want and stop everything a few days or weeks before the contest or take a different drug that's in and out of their body in twenty-four hours. In addition, they can take a few drug masking agents and pass the test with flying colors. Also, do you remember that testosterone/epitestosterone ratio we talked about earlier in this chapter and how the normal ratio is one-to-one and WADA will fail anyone over a four-to-one ratio? Almost every event that claims "testing" will allow up to a six-to-one ratio.

Random Polygraph Testing: Several of these contests rely on polygraph testing to detect drug use by their contestants with absolutely no urine or blood testing. They're all used to lying anyway so the polygraph won't pick up anything. And who exactly is monitoring and evaluating these polygraph tests? As you may have guessed, there's no mention of that either.

Limited Testing: This is testing for certain steroids, but not pro-hormones, SARMs, or other hormone enhancing drugs. And the testing is done only during the contests and at no other times. It states right there on several websites that they will only randomly test for certain things, but everything else is OK to take. I told you it was a joke.

The All-Natural Contests: All of these so-called natural contests say they test for all drugs and that each contestant has to be drug-free for seven years. Some even claim urine testing for all contestants on the day of the contests, but as I mentioned earlier, there are several ways to get around this too. Other contests use polygraph testing or maybe even random (as in never) drug testing. Yeah, that'll keep these contests all natural. And to make these contests have the look of truly being drug-free, they say they follow the WADA list of banned substances. But again, there's no mention of how and when they test, which is basically never. And just like the shows they're promoting, they're all naturally fake.

Back in the early 2000s, I knew a boyfriend and girlfriend who both competed in bodybuilding and fitness contests. I remember watching their bodies drastically change as they got closer to a contest, and no matter how many times people questioned them about drug use, both of them strongly denied taking any kind of drug, even though it was glaringly obvious they were. And to top off their defense, they would always say that all the contests they entered strongly test all contestants for drug use. One day as I was walking into the locker room at the gym, he was walking out in a hurry. And on the floor by a locker were several pre-loaded syringes, a vial of some kind of liquid, and a small towel in which he had obviously wrapped everything to keep it hidden. Because I liked the guy, I ran out and grabbed him and said, "I think you left something in there." His face turned white—and I mean white— and he ran back into the locker room in a panic. When he came back out, he came up to me and said, "Thanks, man. Please don't tell anyone about this." I told him I wouldn't, and later that day he came back up to me. He asked me again to please not tell anyone what happened, and after I told him I wouldn't say a word, I asked him one question. I said, "Just tell me how you and your girlfriend get away with taking steroids if these contests truly test everyone." He said, "It's a big joke. Most contests don't test anyone. They just say they do. And the ones that do test, they do the testing themselves and never bring up the results. Even the judges are on the stuff so nobody really cares anyway."

Drug testing in these events is obsolete, ineffective, and quite comical. And as you can see by the look of the contestants in these events, they have not one worry about getting tested. What about other fitness events and games? Do they test their contestants?

Fitness Games: You've seen these on TV, and just like the bodybuilding and physique contests, the roids are rampant and the testing will just make you laugh. From lifting huge balls of concrete and throwing barrels over a wall, to dropping barbells and flopping around on a chin-up bar, contestants are juicing up to get the win. And as far as testing for steroids and other drugs, it's all random, with some contests saying they test their athletes both in and outside of competition. Again, random is a wide-open term, and in my opinion it's a complete waste of time because everyone knows how to pass these tests anyway. The steroid detector would be working overtime at these events. And the lists of drugs these men and women are taking—you almost feel sorry for their kidneys and livers. All-natural contests? Right! All-natural liars. How about fitness models? Do companies test the models they use in magazines and fitness advertisements? You know, to make sure everything is on the level?

Fitness Models: Ha! Testing models for steroids and other drugs? The only concern companies and ad agencies have about their models is that they look the part. That's it! They have no need and no time for testing. Besides, it's completely irrelevant; all they want is their models looking good. How their models get there is not a concern. And I bet there is even quite a bit of suggestive drug use in this industry; what do you say? What about traditional models we see in magazines and on the runways? Yep, same thing. Look the part or move on. What you see all over fitness advertisements is not what you get, period! I'll get into this in the next chapter so you can see how big the entire fitness scam really is. What about college and professional sports? Are the athletes we see on Saturdays and Sundays subject to drug testing as well?

Professional Sports: Testing among professional sports varies from one sport to another, but this is how the big boys are tested. In professional baseball, every player is tested during spring training and then again later in the regular season. MLB also performs random testing throughout the season. The NFL tests every player at the beginning of training camp and administers random tests on all teams throughout the season. They also test their prospects at the combine. The NBA tests its players randomly throughout the season, but they do not test everyone like the NFL does. The NBA has been criticized often for its gaps in testing. How about the NHL? They also perform random testing, but only a few players have been busted over several years; does that tell you anything? Professional tennis has its testing problems too, and from what I can tell, most of the tests they give are to the top-tiered players only. It really doesn't matter how these different sports test their players for drugs because the players have gotten way too good at passing the tests. What about college players—are they subject to steroid testing as well?

College Athletes: The NCAA has a drug program where it performs random urine tests on student-athletes throughout the academic year. Athletes are notified one to two days prior to testing, but as you'll soon see, this is plenty of time to hide the evidence. Take a minute and think about the last time you heard about a college athlete getting caught using steroids. Exactly! It very rarely happens.

As you can see, drug testing from one end of the fitness industry to the other is more of an appeasement than a solution to stop drugs. There are plenty of claims from all areas of sports and fitness contests of stringent drug testing and efforts to keep the integrity of drug-free contests, but it's all highly questionable. At the end of the day, no amount of testing really matters anyway because drug users have kept up with the pace set by drug testing methods and protocols. You see, they've figured it all out. They know exactly how to beat the system and pass any and every test they may be given.

From peeing in a cup, to giving blood, to taking a polygraph, it's all the same to these professional liars because they have the means and methods to get past any and all testing thrown their way.

I've hinted at a few of these cheating ways, and now I want you to see exactly how they cheat. When I said bodybuilders and fitness contestants know how to cheat a drug test, I wasn't kidding. From powdered piss, to fake dongs, to dehydration, the methods of cheating have no limits. Take a look at my Lab of Lies and see for yourself.

Lab of Lies – Cheating the Test

Self-Testing Kits

This is the first item on the drug cheat sheet, and it allows athletes and contestants to see if the drugs they are taking will be detected. If the drugs do show up then they can start the process of masking these drugs with the other methods I'll talk about shortly. They

---

can also start reducing the drugs they're currently taking and start taking different drugs like testosterone suspension or HGH, which only stay in the body for twenty-four to seventy-two hours. They can use these self-testing kits as many times as they need to until the drugs are completely undetectable. How about that for a cheating start? If drugs are still showing up, or they just want to be extra cautious of not getting caught, they can proceed to the next stage of fraudulent manipulation: powdered urine.

Powdered Urine

It's exactly what it sounds like: dehydrated urine. And as far as availability, you can get it online from countless websites or even in some stores. Go ahead and Google powdered urine and see what pops up; I was surprised at the availability of this stuff.

On the website *Testclear.com*, I found a prime example of a powdered urine kit: "The synthetic urine kit looks, smells, and behaves chemically as drug-free human urine. This gives you complete confidence knowing that the fake pee is able to meet the requirements no matter the sophistication of the experiment."[10]

By experiment they mean test. Most of this fake urine comes in a kit that includes the powdered urine itself, holding bags, vials to hold the fake urine after water is added, heating bags, and the best part of all: a fake dong. I'm not even kidding. These kits even come with detailed instructions on how to get things flowing without getting caught. But there is a drawback to using fake urine: If a person has to give a urine sample while an official is watching, this method is usually abandoned for something more secretive, and it involves the use of a catheter. Ouch!

Using a Catheter

Some contestants call this method foolproof. Really? So I guess it's *unfoolish* to put someone else's urine into your body by way of a catheter? But considering everything else these people put in their bodies, it makes sense. This method is done by inserting a catheter into the urethra and into the bladder and transfusing someone else's urine into one's own bladder. Yep, this really goes on. Never mind the chance of a serious infection; they'll get by with their cheating ways; that's all that matters to them. From my research, many athletes—especially Olympic athletes—use this method. There were even several urine drug tests taken from Olympic athletes that were determined as being the exact same urine. This simply means there were several athletes who got their urine from the same person. I also found where selling your own urine for this exact purpose can net some good money. I guess you could say the urine buyers were definitely pissing away their money.

Blood Transfusions

I mentioned this in the previous chapter when I talked about blood doping and the use of EPO (erythropoietin) to increase red blood cells and oxygen in the blood, but it's definitely high on the list of cheating choices among athletes and other fitness sports contestants. Believe it or not, there is even talk of gene doping, but for now it's all talk. I wouldn't be surprised one bit if it does become the next big thing in performance enhancing drugs. How about that little bottle of soap at your kitchen sink? Can it help competitors cheat their drug tests as well?

Soap-a-pee-ya

That's right, good old bar soap, dish washing detergent, or any household cleansing soap can completely destroy the banned drug EPO in a drug sample. Most soaps contain an enzyme called protease, which destroys EPO and therefore can be added to urine to completely remove any evidence of using EPO. Unbelievable isn't it? And if a competitor still needs to clean more drugs out of their body before testing day, they can try to wash them out with diuretics.

Diuretics

As I mentioned in the last chapter, diuretics simply increase urination and therefore rid the body of as much fluid as possible. They also rid muscle and other tissues of chemicals; this is where diuretics become a masking agent to hide drug use. Remember all of those steroids we talked about in Chapter 3? Each and every one of them causes water retention, and with the exception of a few like suspension and HGH, they are detectable in urine for as long as two to three weeks after last use. And although taking diuretics is extremely dangerous and can lead to life threatening situations, diuretics are the go-to drug for masking steroid use in all of sports and fitness. It's just another way to cover up the lies in a dysfunctional fitness industry, and the price the user has to pay is irrelevant. Do you want to really be blown away with yet another way of cheating we would never think about? OK, here you go. You can put it in ink!

Tattoos

Are you saying, "WTH?" I did too, but here's another big reason competitors are getting inked up. It has been found that taking drugs through tattoo needles increases the effectiveness of steroids, vaccinations, and other drugs. Because the effectiveness is increased, a much lower dose of drugs is needed; therefore, they're harder to detect. I can see the advertisements now: Buy a tattoo and get your steroids 50 percent off! While supplies last of course. Fricking crazy!

Injecting Epitestosterone

Do you remember talking about the testosterone/epitestosterone ratios earlier? WADA says anything over four-to-one will be deemed as a failed test, and further testing would be done. To keep this ratio at or below the accepted four-to-one, athletes and competitors will inject epitestosterone to level out this ratio. And then all they have to do is use those self-testing kits I talked about early in this section to see if their ratios are acceptable. Great plan, right? The losers win again.

Other Ways to Cheat

Although the cheating methods I've mentioned so far are the most widely used, there are other ways that will make you shake your head. It's been known that athletes use what's called Therapeutic Exemption to be allowed to use Ritalin and Adderall to enhance their performance on the field or court. These drugs are for Attention Deficit Hyperactivity Disorder (ADHD), but they are commonly used in much different ways in sports. It's been noted that the use of these ADHD drugs can indeed give an athlete a competitive edge by sharpening reaction times and concentration ability while decreasing fatigue. This is why ADHD drugs are listed on the illegal substance list with WADA. I do want to say that there are definitely some athletes who need ADHD medication to function better in their lives, but the reports of those who don't need it and take it for a sporting advantage are common. Another crazy way to cheat is to combine the drug Viagra with nitrous oxide to increase the flow of oxygen in the bloodstream. Can you imagine the combination of these two drugs? Never mind. That's another book.

The problem with drug testing in sports and in the fitness industry is that testing is obsolete. It's like testing kids in a school where a few students have found a way to get the test answers and then they pass them around or sell them to all the other students. The students never worry about failing a test because they always have the answers. And the bigger problem is that these students will graduate with fake diplomas representing fake educations, and colleges and companies will call on them based on their fake grades.

The fitness industry is no different; we have fake trainers and a bunch of fake fit people posing as something healthy, when they're really nothing but inflated fictitious frauds.

But the testing will continue, and organizations of these so-called fitness events will claim and boast that they are the titans of testing and all of their contestants are drug-free. And again, they're all full of it. The trouble with fitness isn't in people's urine; it's in their lack of integrity and character. And just like steroids, this cowardice is everywhere and it's thriving like crazy. You don't have to go to a bodybuilding or physique competition to see it either; all you have to do is look at social media, at the TV, or open a magazine, and the masquerading muscle is there in all of its glory. All it takes is a little smoke, a few mirrors, and some clever advertising, and millions of people every day fall for the oldest and longest living scam ever: fake fitness.

6 The Hidden Truth Behind Smoke, Mirrors, and Masquerades

What would you guess is the number one selling fitness product of all time? Was it something attached to Jack LaLanne, Suzanne Somers, or Jane Fonda? Nope. What about the in-home exercise craze pushing insane workouts that burned through the fitness market like wildfire over the last ten years—is this the top seller? Not even close. Or maybe it's some kind of food processor, blender, or weight-loss program selling fix-all healthy lifestyle solutions with staged audiences and applause. That's a big NO! OK, so what is it? I'll tell you what it is, but I've got a story for you first.

When I was in high school, I was in Future Farmers of America, where I raised animals all year long and then sold them at an annual sale in the spring. I chose to raise steers and lambs, and during my senior year, I decided to throw turkeys into the mix. I loved raising all of these animals, but as with a lot of things, there was a lot of dirty stuff my mom and I had to deal with. The worst thing about raising these animals was that no matter how careful I was, I always got excrement on me, and let me tell you, it smelled horrible! It didn't matter what I wore or how careful I was about where I stepped, something stinky and nasty was going to end up on me. And whatever got on me ended up getting in the car and the house too, so the smell was everywhere. Have you ever stepped in dog droppings and not known it until you tracked it into your house before you smelled it? This is how it was every single day, but the thing was, I pretty much got used to it. You see, it was all part of the experience, and we just accepted the fact that some was going to get on us in some way; it's just the way it was. And there you have it—the very thing that stunk up everything in sight during my four years of raising livestock, lambs, and turkeys is the very thing that is the number one selling fitness product of all time. You can call it BS or whatever you want, but the truth is, what's hidden behind the smoke, mirrors, and masquerades of selling fitness products flat-out stinks. And you don't even have to get it on you to smell it.

As if incompetent personal trainers and gyms full of drugs weren't bad enough, the fitness industry has yet another means to con its way through your money, your health, and your hopes. From deceitful disclosures, to manipulative misrepresentations, to flat-out false advertising, the fitness industry is pulling off scam after scam by offering amazing, one-of-a-kind, super breakthrough products, all while backing them up with empty promises and gag worthy guarantees. As of now, you may not be able to tell where the smell is coming from, but after I show you how fitness advertisements hide their stinky truths, you'll be able to recognize the source of the stench from a mile away. Fitness advertisements are full of it, and their dog and pony shows have turned into rats and roaches rodeos because when you turn the lights on and expose them, they all scatter into dark and concealed corners. The pomp and circumstance, the lights and cameras, and the smoke and mirrors make fitness products look amazing, but I'm about to pull back the curtains and blow the lid off this whole masquerade.

I'm going to begin this chapter by exposing the dubious and deceitful disclosures used in fitness advertisements. And then there are the products themselves—the wonder workouts and miracle machines we see advertised on a daily basis all over social media and TV, in magazines, and over the radio. Yep, I'm going to show you what most of these are good for too; do you have a fireplace? And what about the models used in fitness advertisements? Are their bodies truly the result of using said products or are their muscle make-overs from something far different? Last, I'm going to put the spot-light on Hollywood and pull back the curtains on how they get their "movie muscle" just in time for their next part.

Fitness advertisements are really nothing more than magic shows; they create illusions of can't-miss health, and people are buying up their products like crazy. In the article, "How to Spot a Fitness Fraud," on *simplefitnesssolutions.com*, author Deborah L. Mullen cited the Federal Trade Commission's statement that "consumers waste billions of dollars on unproven, fraudulently marketed, and sometimes useless health care products and treatments," and went on to advise readers to "avoid the lure of fitness-product charlatans and increase your skills at making educated buying decisions. Try not to buy the hype and stick to 'if it sounds too good to be true, it probably is.'"[11]

I hope that after reading this chapter, you'll start to see right through the endless misleading advertisements and avoid the unpleasant smell that comes from most fitness products. Let's start with what I call Deceitful Disclosures and watch the fit-less lies grow from there.

Deceitful Disclosures

The Disappearing Ink

I know you've seen the ant-sized fine print in advertisements way down at the bottom of the screen, but as far as reading it, you'd have to get really close to your TV and be able to read like a bar-code scanner to catch exactly what that fine print says. Or you can do what I've done and record a commercial or infomercial, play it back, and pause it when the tiny print is flashed. Just in case you haven't been able to see exactly what this print says, I've written a few of them here just for you. There are other things they say, but these are the most common.

- The results we're showing from using this product aren't typical, and you should not expect these same results.

- The people in this program also followed a strict diet and exercise program in conjunction with using this product; do not expect the same results.

- Along with using this program, participants followed a medical weight-loss program. You should not expect the same results.

- The people in this program had lost weight and had been following a regimen of diet and exercise prior to starting this program.

Most of the fitness advertisements I've seen say, "You should not expect the same results." If their products work so wonderfully for everyone as they say, why would they need to disclose this? It's simple; they know their product is worthless, and they don't want to get sued. That's it. At the same time, it sure is funny how fitness commercials portray and emphasize that their product alone will do the trick. Trick is definitely the right word, but the consumer is on the wrong side of it. Now, what about the BS promises of superfast, can't-miss results?

Super-Sonic Success

If you notice, most everyone in fitness advertisements has superfast success, and supposedly you can too for three easy payments. Fitness advertisements prey on the consumer's desire to get fit fast. And not just fast, but super-fast, so they show how their products helped thousands of people who had "tried everything before and nothing worked." And they love showing the overnight success stuff like stomach wraps, magic weight-loss drinks, and, of course, the "I lost five pounds in one day" BS. Here's a rule of thumb about these advertisements: If any advertisement, especially with fitness products, promises fast results, LOOK OUT! Oh, they'll take your credit card in a heartbeat and offer a money-back guarantee, but once you buy it, it's yours, baby, and it will more than likely end up right there by the treadmill you never use. At least you have a thirty- to sixty-day money-back guarantee to return it. Or do you?

Guaranteed Garbage

Yep, they all offer a money-back guarantee with no questions asked if you don't like their product. This is all part of the scam because companies know the chances of anyone going through the trouble of mailing back the products are extremely low. Be aware; there's invisible ink with these money-back guarantees as well so read carefully. If you look really close when these fitness commercials start flashing their money-back guarantees on the screen, in tiny print it will say "minus shipping and handling" or the shortened version, "minus S&H." So it's not a complete money-back guarantee after all. HUH! Watch out for the "buy now" prompts too; they know exactly how to push your buttons.

Pushing Your Buttons

This is probably the best trick companies use to get you to buy now: "But wait! If you order now, we'll throw in a bonus DVD; that's another $30 value, and it's all yours if you order now. But that's not all! For being a valuable customer, we're going to add this healthy cookbook, all for three easy payments of $39.95." And then there's the granddaddy of them all: "For the next one hundred callers, we're going to throw in two more bonus DVDs. That's right! That's another $60 value all for calling now." They act like they're losing money by throwing in all of the "free" stuff, but believe me, it's all worked into the price, and they are making a killing.

Look, their number one goal is not to make you healthy;
it's to make them money. Remember that!

From infomercials to social media selfie stupidity, fitness products are advertised around the clock with no rest times, and their deceitful disclosures always back up their super-fast results. They'll flash their one-of-a-kind products and their tricky testimonials to get you to buy everything from protein powders to weight machines until you get smart and unsubscribe. But there's always TV, radio, and magazines where they can flood you with their fake fitness frenzies. And the actual products they're selling—they've got exactly what you need, and boy are they special. Wonder workouts and miracle machines are just a credit card away, and if you order now, you'll lose five pounds just for lifting your phone. Let's take a closer look at how fitness companies lie their way into your pocketbook by selling workouts and equipment with a sleight of hand and magic dust.

Wonder Workouts and Miracle Machines

How can it be that *everyone* has the best workout ever? Or someone always has this one-of-a-kind exercise machine, that's patent pending of course, which practically does the workout for you. And both the workouts and the machines will give you never-before-seen results, and within a short amount of time, you'll look just like the people in the infomercials and in the videos on social media. Remember when I said that sh*t is the number one selling product in all the world? Advertisements of wonder workouts and miracle machines are where the biggest piles are made; I'm talking about piles of money and piles of something else. What about the wonder workouts that claim ultimate fitness can be yours in just a few months or in only minutes a day? Is there any truth to these, or are they just another source of the bad smell?

Wonder Workouts

You've seen these workouts advertised and the rah-rah fake audiences that go with them, oohing and aahing and clapping when prompted by the audience maestro. The whole act behind these workouts is staged and the exercisers are pre-fit for the part as they all tell you, "It's the best workout I've ever done!" These can't-miss workouts range from the "90-day go hard or go home/beast mode" workouts to the "20 minutes to muscles" workouts, and every single one of them will tell you they are the answers to your fitness woes. Let's take a closer look at these different types of wonder workouts and see how their lame lies leave you looking for results in all the wrong places while they put millions in their pockets.

Go Hard or Go Home/Beast Mode Workouts

According to these types of workouts, ninety days is all you need to totally transform your body to look just like the people in the infomercial. The good news is, you don't even need a gym. I do agree you don't need a gym to get a great workout, but to have the body you've always dreamed about, as they put it, you're going to need a lot longer than ninety days—a lot longer. I guarantee you the people in these infomercials and videos have been working out a heck of a lot longer than three months. I'll talk more about this coming up.

Another truth about these types of workouts is that they are breeding grounds for injuries. The people in these infomercials sure do know how to say "beast mode" a lot, but do they know how to say rehab? In fact, a very popular fitness celebrity from one of these ninety-day hardcore workouts suffered a major injury and had to have surgery. Hmm, I wonder how that happened to such a strong and fit person. It happens all the time with these workouts. Look, I can completely understand the attraction of these types of intense workouts, but you have to be smart about them. And when you take a person who hasn't been working out or someone who has been doing very little in terms of exercise and you throw them into one of these intense workouts, trouble and a future full of surgeries is on the way. Just about all of these workouts are about beating up the body—not making it healthier—but the way they're portrayed and advertised, you'd think they were the best things ever. Not only are they not the best, but also, for the most part, they're the worst.

If you're dead set on doing these types of workouts, listen to your body. If you're having prolonged soreness and joint pain, stop altogether or greatly reduce what you're doing. Also, make certain to take heart rates throughout your workout and know what your safe heart rate ranges are. And last, avoid the riskier movements like jerking weights around, lifting barbells over your head in fast jerky ways, and making yourself throw up. What about those twenty-minute workouts—can you really get all ripped up in the amount of time it takes to take a shower?

20-Minute Muscles

What's really funny to me is that the same companies that make most of the ninety-day programs with hour-long daily workouts are the exact same companies that come up with the twenty-minute workouts too. In addition, they tell you that you do not need to work out an hour a day; all you need is twenty minutes. Really? Then why were they telling everyone that their daily hour-long workouts were exactly what they needed to do to get ripped up and rock hard? So which one is it: an hour a day or twenty minutes a day? That's a pretty significant variation; someone's not being honest. No way! Not in the fitness industry! Everyone is honest when it comes to health, right?

I actually think you can get a lot done by exercising twenty minutes a day, but it's more about maintaining your health than having a ripped and muscular physique. I truly believe that if someone did the right kinds of exercises the right ways and included resistance, cardio, and stretching, they could indeed live a healthy life by exercising twenty minutes a day, as long as they had a healthy diet. But the twenty-minute programs I see being advertised won't get you looking like the models in the commercials, but that's exactly what they want you to believe. Remember what we've already talked about: The people you see in these advertisements are professional models, and they show up fit and ready to lift because they exercise a lot more than twenty minutes a day. And there's something else in their bag-o-fitness that's helping them out. Overall, I think these twenty-minute workouts are fine as long as your expectations are realistic. Some fitness companies are so smart they've figured out that if they keep lowering the amount of time a workout takes, people will really like it and they'll buy it. Remember the eight-minute abs workout? It's inevitable that this eight-minute-long workout will be trumped by a seven-minute workout and then a six, five, and so on. Before long, it'll be the one-minute ab workout that's flying off the shelves.

1-Minute Abs

I can't help but think about the movie *There's Something About Mary* when I hear a commercial for an "abs in minutes" fitness program. There's a scene in which Ben Stiller's character is in the car with a hitchhiker he just picked up, and this guy is telling Stiller about his brand-new exercise program idea, "7-Minute Abs." Stiller's character responds by asking the guy what he thinks would happen if someone came up with "6-Minute Abs." And then the hitchhiker freaks out and gets really mad.

This is exactly what goes on in the fitness industry with these supersonic results workouts. Someone, somewhere is always reducing the minutes it takes to get fit, and presto, another brand-new workout is born that's better than all the rest. Before long there will be a "1-Minute Abs" workout; you wait and see. This is the perfect example of what I said at the very beginning of this book: The fitness industry preys upon the hopes and dreams of those wanting to look and feel better by lying and misleading them with a bunch of BS. Speaking of misleading BS, what about those miracle exercise machines and amazing pieces of exercise equipment you see all over TV and social media—are they putting off a funk too?

Miracle Machines

I'm not sure which piece of exercise equipment makes me laugh harder—the one you hold in your hand and shake back and forth, or the one you wrap around your midsection that's supposed to pump and flex the fat right off of your abs. I'm going to go with the shake thing because it's absolutely hilarious to watch the people using it in the commercials. The faces these people make when they're shaking this thing back and forth—it's like they're either having a baby or they're constipated. The people using this thing had to feel really stupid, but at least they're all muscular, fit, and trim, right? From fancy treadmills and ab machines, to vibrating dumbbells and chin-up bars, exercise equipment commercials want to feed you bad information on building muscle, take your money, and run. Some of the exercise equipment they're selling is actually pretty good, but the way they're selling it stinks of deceit. And then there are pieces of equipment that are better suited as gag gifts or for your kid's toy box than to actually use for exercise. As much as I'd like to rate these "miracle machines," I'm going to pass because that's not what this book is about. Instead, I'm going to break them down into a few categories and show you what they're really good for.

Cardio Kings and Weight Machines

You've seen the fancy treadmills that will take you on journeys all over the earth and the all-in-one home-gym exercise machines, right? Let's start with these. This category is actually where the good stuff is, with most of the treadmills, stair climbers, and stationary bikes being pretty good deals, and the multi-station weight machines offer a good value as well. I think they all make good sense if someone is actually going to use them instead of stacking clothes and Christmas decorations on them in the spare bedroom. You know what I'm talking about. The problem with this type of exercise equipment typically isn't its quality; it's the way the equipment is presented in the infomercials. Yep, here we go again with promises of "Your Best Body Yet," and all you have to do is use this amazing piece of exercise equipment and the magic will happen. And, of course, the models using the showcased exercise machines are lean, ripped, and smiling like they're having fun.

Before you buy one of these cardio or weight machines, make certain you're actually going to use it, do your research on its dependability, and check the many used pieces for sale in various online sales sites for a better price before you pull the trigger. Another thing for you to consider is to make certain of the warranty and repair policy with these machines. Some of the repair costs can be outrageous, which won't be mentioned or disclosed within the infomercial. And last, don't expect to get your brand-new body to show up any time soon like the infomercial tells you it will. Buy the new machine because you like it and you want to add variety to your exercise program, but don't buy it because of the insta-fit body it promises you. What about those pieces of exercise equipment that vibrate and are supposed to practically do the work for you? Are they worth a second look?

Bad Vibrations

You're better off exercising on top of your washing machine or chasing a wind-up toy than buying a piece of exercise equipment that promises your best body through vibrations. Oh, they make it sound like using vibrating exercise equipment is a huge breakthrough and that creating an unstable grip or footing or vibrating your abs is going to help you build your best body ever. In terms of rehabilitation, standing on a vibrating platform while exercising can be beneficial, but beyond that, it's just another heartless lie. This just proves that through the smoke and mirrors of marketing, companies can make mud look good to a river, and the river will buy it up. This type of exercise equipment doesn't work; it's as simple as that. And all of those miracle ab machines being paraded around on the infomercial highway are even bigger "waists" of time.

Abnormalities

From one abdominal machine to the next, promises of a six-pack from using one of these ab-blasting pieces of exercise equipment are made all across late night TV, and apparently millions are falling for it. Everyone wants a six-pack, or at least a four-pack, and fitness equipment companies know this and prey on it. And these companies make their ab machines look all scientific with their "thermal heat-seeking technology" showing how the abs are "heating up" on one of their ultra-fit models as they use their mid-section marvel. I laugh every time I see one of these infomercials pushing an ABsolute piece of crap abdominal machine, especially when they go to a beach or park and have a "stranger" use the machine. And it never fails; the "stranger" always has a response like, "Oh my gosh, this is awesome! I can feel my abs burning, and I don't even feel like I'm exercising. I'm in the gym seven days a week working on my abs, and I've never felt anything like this before." Oh man, now that's funny. But again, for some reason, people believe this nonsense and rush to give their credit card numbers because they want to be one of the first one hundred callers and get two ab miracles for the price of one. Even if they were both free, the customer would end up on the losing end of that deal. And finally, what about those knee, elbow, and back braces in all the advertisements—do they really help with pain, or are these companies lying like everyone else just to make a buck?

Bogus Bracing

Here again is a perfect example of how a fitness product company lies and misleads consumers into buying their products. You've had to see at least a few commercials about these wonder braces for painful joints. You know, where they break out the thermal heat-seeking technology that makes the joints of the body glow bright red to indicate pain, and then someone puts on the wonder brace and, presto, the glowing red color is gone and so is the pain. The truth is, compression braces do help with soreness and inflammation, but they are not going to heal an arthritic joint. When the brace comes off, the pain will return. Compression has been used since the beginning of time, and these companies selling these braces act like it's a whole new discovery. Examples of these products that stand out to me are the braces that have copper in them. The advertisements claim that the combination of compression and copper will heal joint injuries, therefore ridding the joint of pain. BS! There is not one single interaction between compression and copper; it doesn't exist.

In the *skeptoid.com* article, "Joint Pain: Scams, Lies, and Exaggerations, Part 1," author Stephen Propatier wrote, "Vendors will often make suggestive claims about the qualities of copper, such as, 'Copper is an essential trace element vital to all living organisms.' That's true, but only as far as we consume copper; wearing copper doesn't provide any nutrition."[12]

And by the way, the copper they say is the magic part of these braces is usually less than 5 percent of the total product. Sounds like they don't believe their own BS.

From bogus braces to junky fitness equipment, the fraud used to get people to buy useless exercise devices runs deep.

Talking about all of this no-good fitness equipment reminds me of a client I trained in her home a few years back. I'll never forget when I first went to her house and she showed me her home gym. I was blown away but not in a good way. She had a few pieces of cardio equipment, which were actually really good, but everything else was mind blowing. It was like her workout room was a super-info-mercial studio with almost every piece of exercise equipment I had ever seen advertised. She knew by my face that I was shocked, and before I could say anything, she gave me her story.

She told me she wanted more than anything to work out and lose the weight gain she had been fighting for the last fifteen years, but she was too embarrassed and uncomfortable to go to the gym. She said she was drawn into fitness infomercials because they made everything look so easy, and they made her feel she could get all the exercise she needed in the privacy of her own home. When I asked her how long she used the exercise machines, she said, "Not long because it definitely didn't feel the way they made it look, and it really didn't seem like it was doing much for me." And then she said something I'll never forget. She said, "The worst part is the infomercials make you believe you can look like the others who are using the same equipment. They even show several before and after pictures of people who had used the same pieces of equipment and it really drew me in. But after using the equipment for three or four weeks exactly the way I was supposed to, nothing changed like they said it would." I told her all of that was in the past as we started our first workout. Six months later, she was down twenty-eight pounds, and by the end of our first month, all of those gimmicky exercise machines were gone. I asked her one day what she did with them and she said, "I put them where they belong: in the trash!"

A lot of fitness companies tell lies, but they're not dumb. They know their chances of selling a worthless piece of junk greatly increase if they make that worthless piece of junk look really good, and more importantly, if they make the people using the worthless piece of junk look even better. Fitness models are in high demand because companies want their fitness products in the hands of the buff and the beautiful, even if these models have never even heard of their product. Yeah, that's right; chances are, the people shown in these infomercials and exercise videos are first-time users of these products themselves, but they're paid to say otherwise. Throw in a little smoke, a few mirrors, and a little makeup muscle, and the scene is set to look like the best workout ever.

Makeup and Muscle

If someone wants to be in a workout video or commercial, they're going to have to show up fit and ready to fake it. When it comes to any kind of fitness advertisement, the instructors are top notch fit, and for the most part, the other exercisers are fit as fiddles too. All because they have been using these breakthrough workouts and doing nothing else. Yeah, right! Here's where it gets funny. What the advertisements fail to tell you is that both the instructors and the other exercisers have been using other workouts, and, more than likely, many of them had never used the workout they are trying to sell you until a few weeks prior to the commercial. And that's only because they had to rehearse for it. I bet you won't find that in any of their disclosures or fine print. Remember those fitness models I talked about in the last few chapters? These are the very people fitness companies hire to be in their commercials because all they have to do is hand them some dumbbells, make their hair look good, and it's lights, camera, fraud.

The workout advertisements you see on TV and social media are just like the movies; the models get makeovers before the shoot to look their absolute best. But what would you say if I told you they can also paint on six-packs and a few other extra muscle definitions to get that cut look? This very thing is done in movies all the time, and when it comes to advertising in magazines or on social media, photo-retouched pecs and abs is the go-to cheat. I've been around cameras and video shoots enough to know that makeup artists can work miracles and can make a person look twenty years younger and even twenty pounds lighter if needed. Speaking of losing pounds, do models change their diets prior to auditioning for a shoot?

Another important tidbit that fitness commercials will fail to tell you is that many of their exercisers and instructors followed very strict diets months prior to shooting their commercial. What? You mean they didn't get this fit using only this workout? I'm shocked! Fitness models audition for these commercials just like actors do for movies, so they have to be fit and ready to go before anyone will hire them. You know, kind of like a head start. Remember those drugs we talked about earlier? I'll be bringing those up here again shortly. Believe me, exercise models are the Barbie and Ken dolls of the exercise world, and they're really good in these advertisements because they've been doing it for a large part of their lives, they look the part, and they're good on camera. They're also really good at making the workouts look challenging, but at the same time, they make it look easy to learn how to do them. So remember when you're watching an advertisement for a fitness product that the people you see are more than likely involved in a whole lot more than what they're advertising. And I guarantee you, companies that advertise these workouts and other products are not concerned one bit about you calling them out on this because they think you'll never know the difference anyway. And now we get to one of the biggest deceptions with fitness advertisements: DRUGS!

We've already covered this in the last few chapters, so I'm going to make this short and sweet. As I've said, drugs are everywhere in the fitness industry, and you can see them in action in commercials, infomercials, and social media ads. These companies act like their instructors and their exercisers are fit solely because they have been using their wonder workout, but by now, you should know this is all a big fat lie. These exercisers (models) roid up just as much or more than anyone else, and they're really good at lying about it too. Remember, where there's competition, there will be steroids, and the fitness model industry is as competitive as anything else. What about those heartfelt testimonials that always accompany fitness advertisements? Should you have your lie detector on for those as well?

Tricky Testimonials

You better put your boots on for this one; it's about to get deep! When it comes to testimonials, there are three main categories: emotional, amazing transformations, and medical. I know you've seen examples of these where it's either someone crying as they tell their emotional story, someone talking about their amazing physical transformation in a matter of weeks, and, of course, the "doctor" in the white coat and stethoscope sitting in an examining room giving their "medical opinion" of why a particular product is so good. I'll break these down so we can get a good laugh at them all.

Tears of Ploy

Playing on the emotions of the consumer is selling strategy 101. All companies use this strategy, but when it comes to selling fitness products, it's the gold standard. They always have someone tell a sad story and then explain how the product they're using completely turned their life around. Believe me, I'm all for someone improving their life and having long overdue success, but companies that use this tactic to sell their wonder workouts or miracle exercise machines are just more examples of an industry full of lies. I've been in this business too long to not be able to spot full-blown BS, and this is a prime example. They get the person to tell their story, with the sad music of course, and as they get going they tear up. And then something wonderful happens! They start talking about how the product they're using turned their life around (key the upbeat music), and their tears float away on the happy cloud and everyone is in fun town now. Theatrics at its best! Here's a great question for you to think about. How many takes do you think are needed to get the exact response (tears and sadness) from the person giving the testimonial? I've seen these done in person and I'm telling you now, it's more than you can count on both hands. How's that for being genuine? Don't be fooled by the tears; they're there to trick you, just like the before and after pictures.

The other emotional tools advertisements use are the before and after pictures. Oh, we know these well, don't we? Man, the fraud runs deep here because of three big factors. First, there's absolutely no way of telling when the pictures were taken. The before picture could have been taken years before or even at a time when the person was at their heaviest or most out of shape. The after picture could have been taken several years after the before picture and after several years of dieting and exercise; in other words, there's no proof that these photos were taken within the thirty- to ninety-day time period of transformation they want you to buy into. Second, in the before picture, the person is always frowning, pale looking, and has an overall unkempt look to them, whereas with the after picture, they are always smiling, tan, and their hair and everything else looks good. Nothing to hide here. And last, the wonderful, deceiving world of photo-retouching. The before picture is typically low quality and low resolution, while the after photo is very clear, bright, and high resolution. Plus, the after picture might include a little more color here and there and maybe even some muscle definition and a leaner midsection; you know, all the things they promise you'll get by using their workout or equipment. And to top everything off, they're going to promise you that you can have everything you've always wanted with your body in a very short amount of time.

Time-Sensitive Transformations

Companies have done their marketing homework, and they know that showing tears and testimonials is a good thing, but showing miraculous transformations in a short amount of time is the cherry on top. Have you noticed that all of the fitness testimonials always include the amazingly short amount of time it took for the unbelievable transformation? "In just two weeks, I lost twenty pounds and four dress sizes." "I used this product for thirty days and lost 10 percent body fat and gained fifteen pounds of muscle." "I've only been using this product for two weeks and already I have ten times the energy, my waist is three inches smaller, and I'm playing with my kids a lot more often."

Fitness companies know we want our fitness now, and when they promise us we can have the body and the energy we've always wanted in a short amount of time, it becomes much more attractive. And then they bring the hammer! To seal the deal with their never-before-seen program or product, they bring in the big guns: the white coats.

White Coat Syndrome

Most everyone believes what a doctor says, even when the doctor's in a commercial. "Hello, I'm Dr. Pantsonfire, and I tell all of my patients to use the super (insert fitness fraud product here). I even use it myself, and I've seen all of the benefits this product promises. The patent-pending process this product uses greatly improves the health of all of my patients and I recommend its use to everyone." And that's about all it takes. Some advertisements even bring out the "chemist" in a lab coat sitting in a fabricated lab with beakers and tubes and such. What's funny is the chemist you see and some doctors are just actors or people they pay to put on a white coat and act the part. I've seen several commercials where they never actually say that the person in the white coat is a doctor; they just assume you'll think it because of how they look. And the hospital setting doesn't hurt either. Some fitness ads only use pictures of doctors when they say things like, "This product is endorsed by medical professionals all over the United States," and "People all over the medical community are using this product for themselves and their patients." But many times there's not one word that actually says doctors approve and endorse the product. The white coat syndrome in fitness advertising is real, and you're right to be scared.

Another way companies use fake medical industry support in their advertisements is by saying their products miraculously stopped pain and actually healed injuries. These are mainly advertisements for the aging population, but they are going strong. They'll show an elderly person who's obviously in pain struggling to walk or perform an activity, and when they use the exercise equipment, brace, or super supplement, everything is wonderful again. Houdini would be proud. You could say this stuff was made for the movies and you'd be correct.

Movie Muscle

The trickery never ends with fitness advertisements, and one thing is for sure: What you see is definitely not what you get. In most ways, the fitness industry is a lot like the movie industry in that everything is one big act. Actors and actresses get all fit for their parts, they use lighting and makeup to make them look even better, and they act their way through one big made-up script. Almost all of these actors and actresses use Botox, fillers, and other means to keep their faces looking young and attractive; do you think they do artificial things to their bodies to get the same effect? Oh yes, and a lot more than you may realize. It's all part of the business and I do get it, but there's a whole world out there that wants to look, feel, and be like the people in the movies, and they do their best to do so. People want the Wolverine and the 300 body, and they think all they have to do is work out really hard using a workout that the celebrities use and eat a really clean diet. Well, guess what? The extremely fit actors and actresses in the movies did a lot more than just exercise and eat healthy to get their movie muscle, but they'll never admit it.

Many actors and actresses get their movie muscle in the same way other people in the fitness industry get theirs: They inject it.

Do you remember when I was talking about HGH (human growth hormone) in Chapters 4 and 5? This is very popular with celebrities because it's super effective and they can afford it. And HGH isn't the only thing hitting the bloodstreams of these actors and actresses. Testosterone treatments are high on the want list too, and I'd be willing to bet there aren't many who do not partake in this "supplementation," even if they don't need it. And the fat-burning drugs—they take them like vitamins. Look at it like this: How big is plastic surgery in Hollywood? Exactly! So why would they stop there? They want it all, and since the competition is so high, the steroids and other drugs get the red-carpet treatment. Most celebrities have a posh, high-profile life, and it's easy to see why most people would want to live like they do, and that's exactly why companies pair their fitness products with easily recognizable figures from Hollywood to give their products that extra shine. I call it the Hollywood Effect.

The Hollywood Effect

From professional athletes to chart-busting singers and big-screen celebrities, fitness advertisements take advantage of the high-profile payoff of having famous faces and bodies paired with their products. They do a really good job making it look like the celebrity is head over heels about their wonderful product, but the real motivation is money. Celebrities don't just pick a product they like and want to tell the whole world they love it; they are merely doing what they do best; they're getting paid to act and, in most cases, lie. Celebrity-endorsed weight-loss products are probably the best example here. You'll see some celebrity on an infomercial talking about how they struggled to maintain a healthy weight most of their life and then just like that, some miracle weight-loss plan helped them get their body and their life back. Please, give me a break! The truth is, they were asked by the company to endorse the product, a back and forth negotiation on payment took place, the celebrity and their agent agreed on a fee, and the commercial full of lies was shot.

Another good example of the effect celebrity endorsements can have on product sales are those miracle exercise machine commercials we talked about earlier. What's funny is watching the celebrity use the product. With a look of awkwardness and uncertainty, they look like a kid who has just learned to ride a bike. They kind of know how to use it, but they're not completely sure about the whole thing. You can flat-out tell they don't use the equipment, but as long as they look good doing it, I guess nobody really cares.

I can't help but think about an infomercial I saw on a TV show that was actually making fun of ridiculous infomercials/commercials! It was an infomercial for this ladder contraption that could be used as a scaffold, a ladder, a platform, and maybe a few other things. The guy showing it was high energy, of course, and he was showing everyone how easy it was to use this super ladder. And right there with him was a lady cheering him on like a cheerleader. He got it all set up like a scaffold and started climbing up to get onto the platform part, and as he was climbing up, he was purposely shaking the whole thing to show how strong and sturdy it was. Big mistake! As he started climbing out onto the platform, it slightly collapsed, and he tried to reassure the woman that everything was OK because the ladder was locked in place. He took one more step, and the whole thing collapsed to the ground really hard, and all I heard was him groaning in pain. Although this particular product has nothing to do with fitness, it still reminds me of celebrities endorsing fitness products they know nothing about and certainly don't use.

Since we were all kids, we've been taught not to judge a book by its cover because it's what's on the inside that counts the most. With fitness advertisements and the fitness industry as a whole, this is the best advice ever. Throughout my career in the fitness business, I've had numerous conversations with clients and entire audiences about how upside-down and skin-deep fitness has become. I always tell people that when they see a fitness advertisement or someone on social media posting "look at me" workout pictures and boasting about their hard bodies and super-hard, "beast-mode" workouts, there's a lot more going on than just exercising and eating healthy. I remember the very conversation I had with a brand-new client of mine. She told me she had struggled with trying to get that "hard-fit look" for several years and had tried many diets and workout programs with little to no success. She had used personal trainers, and had even gone so far as to join a highly intense exercise program where she ended up getting hurt and wasn't able to work out at all for several months. She was definitely frustrated, and I could tell by the look on her face and the hopeless sound in her voice that she was to the point where she was going to throw her hands up and quit trying if something good didn't happen fast. And one thing she kept saying was that no matter how hard she tried or what she did, she never ended up looking like all the other fit people she saw. She said, "I did the exact things everyone told me to do, and I followed their eating plans, and I never even came close to looking like they did. I feel like I'm just not made to have that fit look, and I hate this feeling. Do you think I can ever be fit like all those other people?" And then I asked her, "What would you say if I told you that almost all of those people you see in fitness advertisements are fake?" She said, "What do you mean?" I said, "Most of those fitness models you see advertising exercise machines, videos, and diet and supplement plans are taking drugs to get their fit look." She said, "No way! They aren't all overly muscular; they're just really lean and fit. Are they really taking drugs?"

I really felt for her because, like so many others out there who put in the effort to look like what our fitness industry has deemed as fit, she was constantly let down because what she was led to believe was going to happen to her body in a relatively short amount of time never happened—over and over again. Here's the rest of what I told her, and I want you to let this sink in real deep:

There's a big difference between what you see in fitness advertisements and reality. Fitness companies are going to make their products look as good as they possibly can by hiring pre-fit models who make working out and being in these advertisements a big part of their lives and have for a long time. They didn't just stumble upon a magic genie and start using some miracle machine or "instant ripped and fit diet plan" and all of a sudden got their amazingly fit looking bodies as these advertisements want you to believe. And most of them cheated. That's right, they took drugs to get that fit look, and if you want to see what I'm talking about, search the Internet for fitness model forums and look at what they are talking about; 90 percent of the conversations are about what kinds of drugs to take and when to take them, with almost nothing about working out. And, as far as those actors and actresses who show up in movies all ripped and buff, they're doing the same drugs as these fitness models, but they'll never admit it. By the way, what do you think they look like when they're not getting ready for a movie? I can tell you they don't walk around all year long with their six-packs and cut bodies; they actually look normal when there's not a movie coming up. One more thing: When it comes down to how we're all going to look from exercising and eating healthy, genetics has the final say-so. We all have genetic predispositions that determine exactly how we're going to respond to different ways of exercising and eating. Just because someone you know gets certain results and can look a certain way from their exercise and diet regimens, doesn't guarantee you will too. But that's OK; it just means we have to find what works best for us as individuals, and sometimes that takes a lot of trial and error. Don't believe the BS from fitness advertisements telling you that all you have to do is follow their plan and you'll be fit too. But at the same time, don't use your fitness challenges as excuses; go find what works best for you and get what you want.

The writing is on the wall with these fantasy fitness products, but you have to read fast to see it because it's gone in a flash. Even though they're forced by law to disclose the truths about their magical products, they still find the loopholes, and with smoke, mirrors, and masquerades, they camouflage these truths really well. Fitness advertisements will promise you steel buns, abs in minutes, and the body you've always wanted in ninety days or less. And if you buy now, they'll throw in instant shoulders and biceps too! And forget going to the gym; you can use their total-body masterpiece or super-slimdown video in your own home to get that rock-hard body in only twenty minutes a day. And when you get sore and your joints hurt, they'll get you all fixed up with their way overpriced joint braces that are made with magic copper and magic dust. The best thing is, you can trust all of these fitness products because the people in the commercials are super fit, their testimonials are heartfelt, and even "doctors" are using the products. And if that's not enough, celebrities are using these products to stay young, fit, and full of energy, so they have to be the real deal, right?

This book is about fraud, plain and simple, and fitness advertisements use a lot of fraudulent means to sell the number one product of all time. You now know what that is, don't you? From walking at the dog park and stepping in a big pile of it, to the endless products sold all over TV and social media, it's all poppycock, and it doesn't end there. Oh, there's plenty more to talk about, and with the endless peddling of snake oils and magic pills from supplement stores and the ever-popular pyramid marketing schemes, more crap is coming. Like I said, be careful where you step; it's everywhere.

7 Avoid the Spiel of Snake Oils, Magic Pills, and Pyramid Power

Step right up! You sir, you look like a strong young man with a good arm. All you have to do is knock these bottles down, and you can choose your prize. Five balls for five dollars and it's easy peasy. Look, I'll even let you in on a secret and show you how it's done.

How about you? I bet I can guess your weight and if I'm wrong, hey, my wrong is your right and the prize is yours.

Ring the bell! That's right, let's see how strong you really are. Ring the bell just one time and any prize is yours!

When I was a kid, the carnival coming to town was as close to Christmas as it could get for me, and even though the carnival always took my money and left me with a stomach ache, I always thought I could come out on top and win a big prize. And I fell hard for those lines the carnies threw at me every single time. They made all the games look so easy as they tossed the softballs into the big tilted baskets, knocked the little furry doll-like things down with baseballs, and picked up the bottle with a string tied to a bamboo stick. And then there were the oversized teddy bears, Sylvesters, Yosemite Sams, Elmer Fudds, Tweety Birds, and other cartoon characters all hanging up in rows directly above the games, so close you could almost touch them. Add the bright lights, the big top, rides, and the smell of cotton candy and corn dogs, and my money was gone in no time. And what did I have to show for it when I left? Cavities and empty pockets.

The carnival is really good at what it does. It lures people in with bright lights, bright colors, circus-type acts, and promises of big prizes, but at the end of the day, just about everyone leaves with a stomach full of junk and a lighter wallet. The real carnival pros weren't the ones running the Tilt-A-Whirl, the Ferris wheel, or the haunted roller coaster ride, no sir. The masters of the midway were the kings of the carnival and the kings of cash. They knew exactly what buttons to push, and they could see a sucker from a mile away. They made a game of chance look like a sitting duck, and all you had to do was give them your money and the prize was surely yours. And when it didn't happen, they would turn into cheerleaders and say, "You almost got it! You're so close; I bet you get it this time," as you handed them another dollar and took your aim. Those carnies made their living convincing people to give them money for a sure thing, when in fact, the chances were slim to none of walking away with a prize and your pride. And the prizes themselves, oh they looked awesome hanging up there under the bright lights for all to see, but in fact, they were cheaply made, and most of them started falling apart even before you made it out of the place. And by the time you actually won something, you had way over paid because you could have bought it for a lot less than all of those five-dollar chances you took.

Games on the midway were and still are one of the biggest and most successful cons going, yet people can't wait to throw their money at them when the carnival comes to town. Believe me, I love carnival games, and I will pay ten or twenty bucks to throw a few baseballs to knock the heck out of those bottles, but it's all in fun, and I don't expect any return on my investment. Any way you look at it, carnival games are a scam, but they're harmless for the most part unless you throw your arm out. Carnival games are one thing, but there's a much bigger scam going on. You don't have to wait for the carnival to roll into town because this scam is putting on its act 24 hours a day, 365 days a year, and they're using the same dubious sales tactics the carnies use. They get your attention by pitching clever words and phrases, making promises of instant can't-miss wins, and showing you how easy it is for you to come out on top with the big prize. And all you have to do is hand over your money. I'm talking about the multi-billion-dollar health supplement business and how the snake oils, magic pills, and multi-level marketing schemes fit right in under the bright lights and cotton candy smells of the midway.

Yes, the BS runs deep here too, and with everything from vitamin A to protein powders to joint pain tonics, the supplement industry is mostly selling the same thing fitness equipment advertisements are selling, and it stinks just as much.

And those so-called "distributors" of the umpteen million multi-level marketing companies out there pedaling pills and potions—they're definitely drinking the Kool-Aid as they turn their social lives into steady streams of relentlessly irritating supplement parties.

In this chapter, I'm going to show you just how big and bogus the supplement business really is, and you'll be shocked by who it is that's running some of the bigger companies. I'm going to show you how unregulated this business is and how companies get away with labels full of lies and what they're hiding in their "proprietary blends." And those "studies" they talk about on their products, wait till you hear what a crock these are. What about multi-level marketing companies and their sketchy sales tactics? I'm talking about the ever-relentless product pushers sharing their residual supplemental sales stories trying to get you in on the ground floor of the can't-miss business opportunity of a lifetime. I'm going to show you why their high pressure sales and overpriced packets of "our products cure everything" are as fake and fraudulent as everything else we've talked about to this point. So just how big is the business of supplements? Apparently not big enough because it's still growing and picking up steam.

Supplemental Income

First of all, when I say health supplements, I'm talking about several things: vitamins and minerals, meal replacements, protein bars, sports nutrition, weight-loss and weight-gain powders and pills, energy drinks, libido enhancers, and anything else you would find in a vitamin or supplement store. Health supplements have always been a big business, but in 1994 the Dietary Supplement Health and Education Act made it grow like wildfire. This act exempted supplements from needing FDA approval of safety and effectiveness before they go on sale. So basically, anyone could take any substance, put it in a bottle, label it, and sell it as a health supplement. That's a real safe thing to do! From that point on, the supplement industry had double-digit growth and practically became a billion-dollar sales industry overnight. I can just see people sitting around a table saying, "So we can take this here cornmeal, a little salt, add a little chopped up peanuts for protein, throw in a little dried squash for vitamins, put it all in a bottle, and sell it as one of those healthy-type supplements for $39.95?" Yep, that's exactly what you can do, and that's exactly what people did and are still doing. How crazy is that?

Today, there are estimates that the health supplement industry brings in roughly $30 to $40 billion a year in revenue. That's a heck of a lot of bottled pills and powders, isn't it? It was plenty big enough for Big Pharma to notice, and apparently, they got tired of watching supplement companies rake in the millions so they either bought out existing supplement companies or started making their own supplements. And since they are all set up with their labs for drug production, they got going pretty fast. In 2009 Proctor and Gamble, a partner of Teva Pharmaceutical Industries, purchased New Chapter, a supplement company that had been around since 1892. Well-known Pfizer bought the makers of Emergen-C several years ago and the pharma giant Wyeth, which made Centrum vitamins and other supplements. To top it off, Bayer, Unilever, Novartis, GlaxoSmithKline, and other pharmaceutical firms all make supplements.

Why is this important?

Because, as the *Fox News* article, "Many Vitamins, Supplements Made by Big Pharmaceutical Companies," explained, "Some people who buy supplements to avoid Big Pharma drug companies may find themselves doing business with Big Herba, instead. Some of the same companies that mass-produce drugs in huge chemical labs also churn out vitamin and herbal pills sold in bottles with rainbows, sunrises and flowers on their labels. However, size does not guarantee quality. Big companies are more likely to seek out bulk ingredient suppliers in less developed countries, said Jana Hildreth of the Analytical Research Collective, a group of scientists advocating better supplement testing. 'They're going to demand lower prices, and with the prices they demand comes lower quality. You basically get what you pay for,' she said."[13]

All supplement companies can put whatever they want in supplements and use their labels of lies to cover up what they don't want consumers to know. Other than a few reputable brands, the chances you're getting exactly what the label says with your supplements is about the same as winning at one of those carnival games—just about zero. And just like those cartoon character prizes hanging nice and high at the carnival games, supplement companies can make their products look like the real McCoy with bright and shiny packaging, adding to the allure of something really good. But when you peel back the label and start seeing what they're not telling you, you'll see the truth behind the trickery and hopefully quit spending your money on a game of chance.

Throughout my career in the fitness industry, I've had many opportunities to produce and sell my own line of supplements, but I never felt comfortable doing it. There's one particular chance I had, and it went like this:

I had been doing personal training for about five years, and a man I knew very well asked me if I ever thought about producing my own line of supplements. I remember my response: "Isn't there enough already?" He laughed and said, "Yes, but you could still have your own line with your name on it." I said, "But how would I make my own? I'd have to buy the ingredients, measure them out, and then bottle them. Doesn't it take a lab for that?" He said, "No, it's a lot easier than that. As a matter of fact, I'm making my own protein powder as we speak, and it's all done in a lab for me. All I do is make a list of ingredients, send the list to them, and they do the rest." My response was, "But how do you know what they're really putting in the bottle? Couldn't they skimp on ingredients or even add other cheaper ingredients so they make more money?" He said, "Yes, but most of it is legit, and the company I use is really trustworthy." He then said something that really set me back. He said, "You can really make things cheap by buying cheaper supplement ingredients like cheaper protein powders and fillers. I talk to the lab every day, and they give me prices based on the quality of ingredients going into my supplements. It all tastes the same regardless of the quality so no one will ever know any way." My response was, "But don't you feel bad that you're selling bad quality supplements?" His response: "It's not bad; it's just not the best." I never produced my own supplements because there's just too much uncertainty about quality and if you're even getting real ingredients at all. No thanks. I'll stick to training.

There are plenty of things supplement companies don't want you to know, and they're certainly not going to disclose them on their labels. So before you throw another dollar down on your next supplement, take a look at my Warning Label, and maybe you'll think twice the next time someone tells you to step right up.

Warning Label

Proprietary Crap Shoot

Oh yes, the perfect disguise. Supplement companies use the words "proprietary blend" or "complex" on many of their labels, suggesting their ingredients are a big secret when, in fact, it's another way to cheapen up the product with less expensive ingredients.

Here's the loophole: The FDA requires manufacturers to list all of the ingredients in a product on its label, along with the amount of each (typically in micrograms or grams), **unless the ingredients are part of a proprietary blend.** If that's the case, then the specific amount of each individual ingredient in the blend does not have to be listed, only the ingredients themselves and the total amount of the proprietary blend as a whole. Basically, companies can really skimp on effective ingredients and instead put a whole bunch of useless garbage in a supplement, and they don't have to tell you anything. Supplement companies will tell you the reason they use "proprietary blend" or "complex" on their products is because they want to keep their blend of ingredients a secret; you make the call. And here we go again with yet another fraud and another reason for me to write this book. What about the licensing and other requirements for selling supplements—can just anyone make and sell them?

Emancipation Regulation

Remember when I told you in Chapter 2 how easy it is to get a personal trainer certification? Things just got even easier! There are absolutely zero qualifications, licensing, or any other require-ments to produce and sell supplements. Even a four-year-old could make and sell supplements if they could muster up the money, and it would be perfectly legal to do so. Ha! Can you imagine a bunch of toddlers walking around with oversized baby bottles full of amino acids? How about protein pacifiers? Or even post-play-period recovery drinks? It's funny to think about, but I guarantee you someone has thought about it. My point is, the production of supplements is 100 percent unregulated to the point they go to market, and when they do get in the market, all a company has to do is prove their labels match their ingredients—that is if they are ever questioned, which is very rare. Or they can simply use the pro-prietary blend loophole. In addition, the steps the FDA has to take to investigate a supplement are quite lengthy and scientific, which costs the government a lot of time and money. It's very similar to the challenges faced with drug testing. Remember those? Even if a company is caught cheating on the ingredients in its supplements, it's very hard to prove in a court of law. So just like athletes and fitness competitors who use drugs, supplement companies aren't afraid of getting caught because of the lackluster ways of testing. If this isn't a scandal, I don't know what is.

Ingredient Roulette

I watch *Bizarre Foods* with Andrew Zimmern, and some of the stuff he eats almost makes me gag. I love the show, and it is interesting how people from all parts of the world prepare and eat their food. I just shake my head at some of the ingredients and am glad I'm not the one who's having to eat it. With supplements, some of the ingredients that companies use to fill out their products can get weird and unhealthy too, and companies do this so their manufacturing costs are lower. And the ingredient amounts they say are in their supplements can be way off as well. As a matter of fact, several companies have been brought up on lawsuits with allegations their supplement labels were greatly exaggerated. And when their ingredients were tested, huge discrepancies were found. Protein powders were some of the more common supplements where big variations were discovered. For example, some protein powders claimed 30 grams of protein per serving, but when they were measured, the amount of protein was barely 15 grams per serving.

One way that supplement companies fudge their protein amounts is by substituting amino acids for protein. Amino acids are not protein; they are building blocks of protein, which is very different. Companies also substitute cheap fillers such as corn, rice, hydrogenated oils, and "other ingredients" to fill out their products. Other or "inactive" ingredients are commonly used in many supplements and are not there for your health. You can typically find these at the bottom of the label on most supplements. Does this make supplements dangerous? Not really, but the supplement industry does have a history of dangerous products that caused critical illnesses and even death before being pulled from the shelves. Is this a case of better late than never? I don't think so.

Banned Too Late

I can think of several bad supplements currently on the market that are anything but healthy, but there are two that were banned several years ago that are beyond bad: GHB and ephedra. You may recall GHB from Chapter 4. GHB resembles ecstasy and was commonly referred to as the date rape drug. This very drug was available in just about every supplement store in the country prior to 1990 when it was banned by the FDA. And even after its ban, it was being produced in garages and homes by the gallons even though it is illegal to do so. Do you remember in Chapters 3 and 4 when I talked about drugs and, more specifically, GHB? And the story of how I witnessed two trainers falling asleep in the middle of their sessions with clients and how those trainers were subsequently arrested? Well, one of the trainers who got busted and sent to prison actually had a storage unit right by the gym where we all trained. It was said by several people close to him that when the police searched this storage unit, they found more than thirty gallons of GHB ready for distribution. If this drug had never hit the shelves in the first place, it might not have become so popular. Many deaths were reported from using this drug—the very drug that was once legal to sell as a health supplement, just like the next drug.

Ephedra was considered the weight-loss gold standard supplement up until its ban in 2004. Did it work? Yes, it did, but it also did other very bad things. Numerous deaths from heart attacks and arrhythmias were reported as a result from taking ephedra, and shortly after, it was declared an illegal drug to sell. To be fair, these deaths from ephedra could have been from overdosing, but either way you look at it, it's probably too dangerous to be on shelves.

Both of these harmful drugs were allowed in the market without any research whatsoever, and before they were pulled from the shelves, the damage had already been done—both to the people taking these supplements and to the FDA for allowing them to be sold in the first place. As you can see, there is much more to know about supplements than what manufacturers reveal on their labels. There are just too many things they don't have to tell you, and even when they do volunteer information about their products, you have to read between the lines and be able to spot the dangers and the phonies. Here's a question for you: Have you ever wondered exactly who it is that makes supplements? Is it the company selling them or is it something far different?

Mystery Manufacturing

With the exception of a select few, many supplement companies have their products made for them by huge manufacturing plants, and the quality of the ingredients is largely determined by the huge manufacturers and not the company doing the actual selling. As the *Consumerlab.com* website explained, "You can try to ask a manufacturer or distributor for the 'country of origin' of ingredients in its product, but it may not be provided. Be aware that manufacturers may change the source of an ingredient over time. Even if you learn that an ingredient is from China—as many are—ingredient suppliers typically sell more than one version of an ingredient, each differing in quality and cost. It is up to the company making the final product to decide what grade of ingredient to purchase and use."[14]

Here's how it all goes down:

- A supplement company decides on the type and amount of each ingredient they want in their supplement.

- If they are not making the supplement themselves, they then contact a manufacturing lab and come to an agreement on the cost of manufacturing their supplement.

- The manufacturing lab then contacts suppliers of the different ingredients and makes a deal for a certain amount of each. The quality of ingredients varies from source to source, and this is almost impossible to know, unless you can get the supplement company to tell you where they get their ingredients.

- The manufacturer then puts all of the ingredients together, puts them in a bottle or other container, puts the supplement company's label on it, and ships it out.

- Some companies have their products tested by a third party before they are shipped but this is not done by most. And as you will soon see, any and all testing methods are subject to scrutiny.

If you take a close look at your supplement bottle or package, you will typically see "Produced for," "Manufactured for," or "Distributed by" on the bottom of the label. All of these phrases typically mean a supplement company did not make their own supplements, but instead had another manufacturer make the supplement for them. Now that the curtains have been pulled back on how most supplements are made, let's turn our attention to research, which companies supposedly spend millions of dollars to implement. Most of these supplement companies will use "scientific studies" and "research proven" as their go-to slogans to gain your attention and trust, but as you will soon see, these words only mean one thing: Buyer beware!

Studies Show

How many times have you watched a commercial and heard the words, "Clinically and research proven," or "Studies show"? These seem to be the standard ho-hum claims of any and all supplement ads, and just about all of them are biased and BS. Hey, that could be the name of a rock band! Now on stage, Biased and Bullsh*t!

These companies want you to think they spend millions of dollars in labs conducting high-end research and experiments with their magic pills, but the truth is, most of this research is like a couple of three-year-olds mixing different colors of PlayDoh and then giggling about it.

There are three main ways companies get their "research" and "studies" information about their supplements: They borrow research already done from other companies; they do their own research; or they pay a third-party research company to do it for them. Any way they choose, it's ultimately up to them what they let you see.

Copy and Paste

Can you say plagiarism? To save a buck, companies will use research that was previously conducted for other companies and slap it on their own supplement products. Presto! It's done! Just like that! It goes on all the time, and as I've said before, who's going to call them out on it anyway? There's a big problem with this though: There are far too many variables. I'm talking about the amounts and quality of the products, the subjects themselves, conditions like temperature and timing, and other variables used by the different companies doing these experiments and research. And what about other ingredients combined with certain supplements—are they going to be exactly the same across the board? I think you get my point. Can you imagine if doctors prescribed your medication based on someone else's blood work, medical history, and symptoms? Copying and pasting research doesn't sit well with me; how about you? They could just do the research from inside the company, you know, so they know it was done right.

Insider Information

"I've got a great idea," said the CEO of a supplement company. "Let's do the research ourselves! We'll save a ton of money, it will be convenient, and we can make the research turn out any way we want." Even though the wording may be different, the sentiment is very accurate. Many of these supplement companies do their own research, which means they hand-pick their subjects, the conditions, and the timing to enhance the desired outcome. The results may turn out just a little bit biased, don't you think? The whole "lipstick on a pig" saying comes to mind here. A company doing its own research is like letting a defendant in a court case choose the entire jury. The defendant would, of course, pick their closest family members and friends so that no matter what evidence showed up, the jury would decide in the defendant's favor. And that's exactly what many companies do. Studies show companies lie!

For example, let's say a company wants to do their own research on a brand-new weight-loss supplement, so they interview several people and pick only those who have considerable weight to lose, have had an easy time losing weight before, who will follow a planned-out exercise routine, and who will stick to a strict diet that the company will provide for them. The company then begins the trial under very controlled conditions of exercise and diet, all while giving the subjects timely dosages of their trial supplement. If the subjects don't lose weight fast enough, the company increases the amount of exercise, tightens up the diet, and in a lot of cases, increases the supplement dosage (which may or may not have any effect at all). And when the subjects lose a considerable amount of weight, STOP THE PRESSES! THE RESULTS ARE IN! And just like that, their proprietary blend, scientifically proven, patent-pending, never-before-seen wonder weight-loss supplement is born! The thing is, the subjects would have lost weight anyway without the supplement because of their frequent exercise and strict diet, and even though they were considerably heavier than they should be, they have a history of losing weight easily. But the supplement company will pitch the results as being due to nothing other than the supplement itself. Bring on the pig again. And what about those not so good findings supplement companies don't want you to know about?

This is another reason companies do their own research; they can control exactly what they do and do not report. Side effects? What side effects? Nausea, headaches, and nervousness? That wasn't from our supplement; that was from something else they took. And what about the people in the study who had no changes at all? Oh, everybody in our study showed amazing results! Right! Believe me, there is plenty that companies aren't telling us about their supplements because they don't have to. What about other variables that affected the study's outcome that will never be disclosed, like when their subjects take other supplements in addition to the one being tested? And hopefully you haven't forgotten about the chapters on drugs. Do you think that companies drug test their subjects prior to conducting their own studies? Ha! Now that's funny! Think about the millions of muscle-building supplements and the commercials that advertise and push them; yep, we've covered this already but it's worth mentioning again. Regardless of the company, if they are doing their own research on a hot new supplement, just know that their results are like Swiss cheese—there's a whole lot of holes. What about third-party studies? Are they more accurate and on the level?

Third Party

Another option companies have for product testing is to hire a third party with no financial or other attachments to the company owning the product. Is this good? It depends. Some of these companies are reliable and trustworthy while others are worthless. Here we go with the roulette again. The trick is knowing which ones are honest and which ones just tell companies what they want to hear about their supplements. These third parties are getting paid so their noses may be a little brown. I wonder which supplement is causing that. It's probably the same one I used to step in a lot when I was in FFA. Here's the skinny: When it comes to third-party research on a supplement, the results will be given back to the company producing the supplement for their own analysis. At this point, the company can do whatever they want with the results. Hopefully they will use the results to make their supplement better, but more than likely, they'll advertise the good findings, if there are any, and disregard the bad stuff. But at least they can say they had an outside source test their products, like that means anything. On the transparent side of things, if a company lets a third-party testing company make the results public without leaving anything out, that's the company from which I'm going to buy my supplements.

Next up, it's time to flex some marketing muscle and make sure the shiny new supplement catches your eye and your money.

Marketing Muscle

Supplement companies and carnivals have almost identical marketing schemes: They both use bright lights, bold colors, and food; and they both promise to make you much better off. But instead of using stuffed animals, supplement companies use the lure of the label and fiery advertisements to catch the consumer's eye. Walking into a health/supplement store is like walking up to a fireworks stand; you can't help but be attracted to the lightning bolts, sparks, and stars. Think about the candy aisle: Candy makers know exactly how to package their goods, and even though none of it is good for us, we buy it anyway. Supplement companies spend countless dollars on marketing basically to out-label their competition. Since very few people know much about supplements, many consumers buy based on how good the label looks. What ever happened to the old saying, "It's what's on the inside that counts"? Apparently, that's not the case with supplements. And then to add to the allure, supplement companies pair their shiny labels with extremely fit models in their advertisements and cha-ching, the dollars start rolling in.

In the previous chapter I talked about how fitness companies use fitness models to push their exercise equipment. It's the exact same thing with supplements. And just like the chances of those fitness models getting their fit bodies from using the advertised fitness machine are zero to none, the same holds true for fitness models and the supplements they're pushing. Some of them may actually be taking the supplements, but as you know by now, the chances are pretty strong they are taking other "supplements" as well. Having extremely fit models in supplement advertisements is one way for a company to flex its marketing muscle, but another very popular way is by using the power of protein.

The Protein Phenomenon

According to most supplement companies, any product that has "added protein" is automatically good for you. I know you've seen the protein cookies, right? Take a long, hard look at those labels and see what you're getting. Oh, they've definitely added the protein, but the other junk is still in there too—sugar, fat, and sodium. As a matter of fact, the total calories were more than likely increased as well, and even though those added calories were from protein, it's still added calories. Other common products I've seen with added protein include flavored popcorn, protein bars, energy bars, and energy drinks, to name a few. Now, it's one thing to reduce sugar and fat and replace them with protein calories, but this is typically not the case. In fact, many food supplements will increase the simple sugar, fat, and sodium when protein is added so the taste is better. The food industry is really good at this too, but we'll talk about that coming up in the next chapter. Typically, with supplements, if it looks good, people will buy it. And if the sales-people are good at their craft, it's almost an automatic done deal. Supplement sales are through the roof, and just like personal train-ers, there's a salesperson around every corner willing to sign you up for a six-pack. Add the luster of being your own boss, promises of financial freedom, and the prestige of being your own distributor, and you've got yourself some full-blown pyramid power!

Pyramid Power: The Holistic Hoax

Supplements are a huge business, and supplement companies and Big Pharma aren't the only ones who want a piece of the action. There's a whole other group that's putting flashy labels on pills and powders and selling them as hope in a bottle. I'm talking about multi-level marketing companies staking their distributor claim on supplement sales. And there are a bunch of them. Estimates show that there are currently twenty to twenty-five million individual MLM distributors in the United States and somewhere around twelve hundred different MLM companies in business today. The actual number of MLM companies is hard to pinpoint simply because there are so many starting up and collapsing at the same time. Either way, that's a lot of folks pushing pills or other stuff they know nothing about. Even though MLM companies are selling supplements just like the other companies, MLM companies put an entirely different spin on the holistic hoax.

In addition to claiming illness cures and superior products like everyone else does, they're recruiting salespeople with promises of quick cash, hefty salaries, and financial freedom, all from their dubious downline.

Do their promises hold true, or are they earning the liar label like most everyone else in the fitness industry? I'm picking the latter.

I can't even count the times I have been approached by someone who is gung ho about their new can't-miss MLM supplement business venture, but it doesn't take long for me to end the conversation. I'm sure most of us have known someone selling supplements or something else "magical" for one of these MLM companies. What's funny to me is that every person involved tells the same old story in their relentless recruiting attempts: There's always someone who's made millions by selling the product, there's a doctor or two at the helm, they have a patent on some magical far-away berry that cures all kinds of illnesses, and you can work from home on your own time. Plus, they always glorify a fortune-making distributor downline that will rid you of your financial woes. Let's take a closer look at each of these claims and see for once and for all how MLM companies coax their hoax.

"Hey man, I've been waiting to tell you about what I'm doing because I wanted to make sure it was real, and it definitely is! Look, I've got a friend who's been making a killing off this new line of supplements. He showed me a check stub for $50,000, and he's making more than that every month. He got in on the ground floor of this brand-new state-of-the-art supplement company that has a patent on this type of berry that can be found only in the mountains of Siberia. It's making people lose a ton of weight, it's giving them crazy energy, and it's even helping a lot of people get off their medications. The doctor who started this company has been doing research for the last five years and nobody else knows about it. He's even collected the berries himself at times. Because he's got the patent on it, every single supplement store will want what he's got, and guess what? You and I can be on the very top of this thing and make millions. You can become a distributor like me and sell these supplements, and all you have to do is sign up and then get others to sign up under you, and you'll make money from everything they sell too. It's a no-brainer, man, and I've already made $2,000 my first week. This guy who told me about it just bought a summer home in Florida, and he's actually having a meeting next week. Come with me, and you'll see how unbelievably good this deal really is. We're going to make millions! Oh, and by the way, bring $200 for your distributor's license."

This is the typical MLM BS sales rant, and although the products vary from scheme to scheme, the rah-rah easy money sales pitch is easily recognizable. And it never fails, the conversation always begins with an opportunity for fast cash and financial freedom.

From Brags to Riches

Most MLM recruiting conversations begin with a financial hook—a story of someone or of multiple people becoming crazy rich from selling their fantastic product. Some recruiters will even say they were shown pay stubs or copies of checks in the tens of thousands of dollars from "the guy who started the whole thing." But the truth is, there is only a very small percentage of people who actually make money within MLM sales. From my research, I luckily stumbled upon the king of MLM scam busters, Robert L. FitzPatrick. During my interview with FitzPatrick, I learned many things I did not know about MLM. First, very few people in MLM companies make any money at all, and in fact, most lose money. In addition, most of the income generated in these MLM schemes is from distributor sign-up fees and the money these new distributors spend buying the products themselves to stay "qualified" to receive commissions, not from non-distributor sales.

In his article, "The 10 Big Lies of Multi-Level Marketing,"[15] FitzPatrick stated that in one of the largest of all MLM companies, only one half of one percent of all distributors make it to the basic level of "direct" distributor, and the average gross income (before taxes and expenses) of all distributors was about forty dollars a month. When expenses are factored in, nearly all suffer a loss. When a state attorney general filed charges against this company, the tax returns revealed an average net loss of $918 for that state's direct distributors. That's net loss! This doesn't surprise me one bit. FitzPatrick also reported that the recruitment into these companies is largely based upon the offer of an "income opportunity," yet statistics show that the income opportunity is essentially nonexistent and falsely promoted. And while the distributors sink deeper into the red, the top 1 percent are still making commissions from distributor fees.

But the dubious downline continues to feed these companies, and "prospects" keep buying in so one day soon, they too can be at the top—the top of horsesh*t mountain.

Dubious Downline

As FitzPatrick stated, almost all income comes from distributor sign-up fees and from their own purchases of the products, not outside (non-distributor) sales. Oh, it all looks great on paper and it seems easily attainable, but reality paints a much different picture. The thought of having hundreds of people in your downline selling this brand-new wonder supplement creates a mathematical fantasy of making hand over fist money, but it doesn't pan out. For one thing, most distributors drop out within the first year, resulting in a 50–70 percent dropout rate with most MLM companies, according to FitzPatrick and other reports. And with the huge drop in distributorship comes a huge drop in product sales, which creates a constant need to sign up new distributors as fast as possible. I wonder how many closets and garages around the United States are stocked high with supplements that distributors bought themselves to stay qualified to get their ever diminishing commissions. I'm willing to bet there are hundreds of thousands who have enough inventory to open their own stores, but for what they paid for their inventories, they'll still end up on the losing end of things. Maybe those berries weren't so magical after all.

Faraway Berries and Miracle Cures

Oh yes, the magical berry or plant that cures everything from diabetes to hair loss. I think a lot of these MLM supplement companies buy books on rare plants, find the rarest ones in the most extreme places, and pick one to be their super plant. It could be a rare flower or some unheard of plant in the deepest of ocean waters, but whatever it is, it's always a substance with super healing, illness curing, or immune boosting powers. And there's always someone who had a miraculous turn for the better with their health, and, of course, they give their new wonder supplement all the credit. Speaking of plants, did you know MLM companies will plant someone in their audience at their recruiting parties to tell some BS miracle healing story from using their supplements? Or maybe they act skeptical and unsure with scripted and planned questions and eventually they become a distributor right in front of everyone. Yep, goes on all the time. You remember what this book is about, right? OK, just making sure. Do you also remember when I talked about how supplement companies use phrases like "studies show," "scientifically proven," and "clinically proven," and how they "test" their supplements? MLM companies do the same fake and super biased testing on their magical beans too, so don't believe their "findings." Look, this is an automatic huge red flashing light when a company says they have this never-before-seen super plant or proprietary blend of ingredients that cures illnesses. And when they tell you it costs so much because they have to go to great lengths to get it from a one-mile-deep cave at the top of Mt. Everest in the dead of winter because that's the only time it grows, it's on you if you believe that nonsense. And the fact that most MLM distributors think and act like they magically became overnight certified nutritionists should be another warning to you that something definitely stinks within the wonderland pyramid.

Overnight Nutritionists

It's as easy as one-two-three! Sign up as a distributor, pay your sign-up fee, and BAM! You're qualified and certified to teach others about the world of nutrition. At least this is what MLM supplement distributors think. You've heard them talk and push their magic beans as they throw in a few scientific terms, a few miracle stories, and, of course, some doctor nobody has heard of. Some of the "advanced certified" ones will even get into how the body digests and absorbs nutrients. I absolutely love hearing someone from one of these MLM supplement companies pitch their products, and it's like Christmas if they pitch them to me. Not too long ago at a trade show I had the privilege of being recruited by a distributor of a "can't-miss opportunity of a lifetime," and the conversation went like this:

MLM: Hello. I see you're a trainer and you have exercise videos.

Me: Yes, I've been in the business quite a while now.

MLM: Do you recommend supplements to your clients?

Me: (To keep the conversation going) Absolutely. I have all my clients take supplements.

MLM: Have you ever heard of (MLM company)?

ME: Yes, but I don't know a lot about it.

MLM: I'm a distributor, and I can get you some samples so you can see how good our supplements are.

Me: Tell me about your supplements.

MLM: We have a patented proprietary blend of the exact amount of vitamins, minerals, protein, carbohydrates, and rare plant extracts that work perfectly with the body, and our products are absorbed ten times better than all other supplements. We have pre- and post-workout drinks, meal replacements, cleansing systems, herbal energizing pills, weight-loss products, and much more.

Me: (Smiling) WOW! You guys have everything. What is it that makes the nutrients be absorbed so much better than anything else?

MLM: It's the amount of each and how they're formulated that makes them work so well. Dr. Nobody did the research himself, and all the studies are being used by major universities. There are even a few professional sports teams using our products.

Me: So you're saying that your company is the only one that knows exactly how much to take and has the processing of its nutrients down so well that they are absorbed ten times better than nutrients from all other companies?

MLM: (Hesitation and nervousness) Well, from our research we feel we have the best thing going in supplements, and we have hundreds of testimonials from people with severe illnesses who have made full recoveries from taking our products.

Me: Back up a minute; you still didn't explain exactly why your supplements are better than everyone else's. Where are your supplements made, and what is the breakdown of nutrients in your proprietary blend? And you said, "Our research;" did you do the research yourself?

MLM: (Oh sh*t moment) I'll have to check on that. I know they're made in the United States, but I'm not sure where. I don't think we have the breakdown of our proprietary blend, but I'll ask a senior adviser. No, I didn't do the research; other people in the company did it.

Me: OK. I'd love to talk to one of your senior advisers. But here's another question for you: What proof does your company have that your supplements were indeed the reason for recovery from severe illness in the hundreds of people who claim this? Also, what were their illnesses, and were they under the care of a doctor and using prescribed medications as well?

MLM: I'm not sure what their exact illnesses were or what their treatment was. But I can research it and get back to you.

Me: I work with many patients who have major health issues, and if I tell them to take your company's supplements, you're guaranteeing me and them that they will get better?

MLM: It depends on if they use it correctly.

Me: Let's just say they use it exactly as directed by your company; will they automatically get better?

MLM: Not everyone responds the same, and I'll have to ask my senior adviser about certain illnesses.

Me: How much are your supplements?

MLM: (Perking up) That's a great question. It depends on at what level you join. You have to be a distributor to sell our supplements, and it's easy to join; you just pay $500, and you automatically get 20 percent off all products for your clients and for yourself. The key is to get your clients to sign up and sell them too. I'll go get you some information.

Me: That's OK, I'm good. I would like to talk with your senior adviser though. Can you send them over?

The guy left, and I never saw him or his adviser the rest of the time there. This guy could not answer any questions beyond the original BS script he was taught to use. He couldn't respond to any question with specific answers, which is the telltale sign of a supplement distributor thinking they are overnight nutritionists. They'll happily tell you how well their products work, but when it comes to explaining in detail why they work, the distributor will dodge, stumble, drop their toy, and run away. With the exception of claiming super flowers with powers, the basic ingredients in most MLM supplements are no different from what you will find in a health food or supplement store, but the quality, research results and claims, and manufacturing sources are all suspect, and you should be very leery. Some of these MLM supplements have quality ingredients, but they are overpriced and aren't going to cure the illnesses of the world, no matter how much they try to convince you otherwise. And just like the carnies, MLM supplement distributors can lure you in and talk you into throwing your money down on a sure thing. And that prize of health and financial independence they shove down your throat won't get you anything but a sour stomach, a feeling of regret, and a never diminishing inventory of pills and powders that sit right beside all the boxes of other stuff you never use.

Supplemental Summary

Overall, I do believe certain supplements play an essential role in achieving good health, but you have to be very careful which ones you buy into. To help you out, I've made a list of things for you to consider before taking the pill or powder plunge; just think of it as your supplement cheat sheet.

- Do your research. Before you buy a supplement, use these resources to check its rating and quality. These sites are unbiased and will give you exactly what you need to know about supplements and their safety.

    - *https://www.fda.gov/Food/GuidanceRegulation/ GuidanceDocumentsRegulatoryInformation/ DietarySupplements/default.htm*

    - *www.webmd.com*

- Look for "proprietary blend" on labels. If you see proprietary blend on a supplement label, I'd leave it on the shelf. As you saw previously, there's just too much a company can hide with this label. Or you can take a picture of the label, call the company, and ask them what exactly is in their proprietary blend. Not just what's in it, but the amount of each ingredient and where they get these ingredients. Chances are, they won't tell you. And there's the only answer you really need.

- Look for transparency. Stick to supplement companies that are completely transparent. This means they list all ingredients and their amounts, they show where the supplement was made, and they will answer any and all questions you ask.

- Stick to the basics. When it comes to supplements, stick to the basic stuff like vitamins and minerals, protein powders, green foods (ground up and dried vegetable powders), essential oils (omega-3, -6, and -9), branched-chain amino acids, and maybe a few healthy herbs. But just because these are basic doesn't mean they're good. Use the information on this list and check them out before you put them into your body. Most of the other stuff like pre-workout energy powders and drinks, libido enhancers, weight-loss pills, weight-gain pills, and other gimmicky supplements are more than likely a waste of your money and your hopes.

The most important thing to remember about supplement companies is that their number one goal is to make a profit. Your health is a very distant second, if it's even on their radar at all. They'll dress up their snake oils and magic pills with lightning bolts and bright colors to make their products look like the easy answers to all of your wellness woes. And they'll boast about their bogus studies that prove the magic is really in their pills and powders.

The only magic with most supplements is when you hand over your cash or credit card in exchange for a bottle of fat chance and better luck next time.

And watch out for all of those distributors who graduated from MLM University with their degrees in ruining friendships and mastering midway games; they'll be happy to show you how you can have a life under the big top as well. But underneath the empty promises of instant riches, illness cures, and ten-hour work weeks is the reality of a less than 1 percent chance of making a profit. Just like everything else we've talked about in this book, the supplement industry is yet another means of turning what's supposed to be a healthy industry into one big holistic hoax. There is nothing about health that should be anything close to a game of chance, but the carnival says otherwise, and we all know how that turns out. The truth is, if you eat the right foods in the right amounts and at the right times, supplements become obsolete very fast. Unfortunately, even when it comes to making good choices about which foods we eat, we have to be very aware of yet another dirty truth in the fitness industry: food fraud.

8 Eating Clean
The Dirty Truth

Saturday morning cartoons and a bowl full of Froot Loops—at six years old, it's all I needed for everything to be right with the world. On occasion, and if I was lucky and not in any trouble for throwing rocks, my mom would make cinnamon toast as I watched impatiently, standing in front of the oven waiting for the golden moment to pull those bad boys out and go to eating. First, I'd scrape all the excess cinnamon, sugar, and butter off with a spoon or fork and eat it, and then I'd go to town on the toast itself. Yeah, I know it was weird but that's how I did it. And then there was the all mighty special occasion breakfast of chocolate bread. That's right, chocolate bread. Basically, it was crumbled up white bread on a plate with a homemade hot chocolate sauce poured over it, which made me both happy and hyper. But there was one more step to complete before I got to inhale the sweet heaven that awaited: I had to pour ice cold milk over the whole thing, which cooled things off a little and made the chocolate sauce really thick. And then stand back; it was game on! We ate other things, like SOS (ground beef and gravy over toast) and traditional breakfasts of bacon, eggs, and pancakes, but I was always in favor of something sweet and crunchy for my first meal, or any meal of the day for that matter. And then one day out of the blue, something terrible happened; the breakfast menu had a big change and my sweet surprises were history.

As best as I can remember, I was about nine or ten years old when the big change happened. Without warning, Froot Loops, cinnamon toast, and chocolate bread were replaced with oatmeal, homemade wheat toast, eggs, turkey bacon, and fruit. I remember thinking, "WTH?" It was my mom who pulled rank and told all of us all of that sweet stuff and other junk food was going to kill us. Her exact words were, "That junk is going to rot your teeth and your insides." And that was that. The only time I got to eat the sweet stuff was when I got to spend the night at a friend's or cousin's house. But my mom didn't stop with breakfast. She started growing her own vegetables and canning them like crazy. She bought a bread maker and started making all of our bread from scratch. Even the peanut butter she bought was the all-natural variety; you know, the kind where the oil sits on top and you have to stir it like crazy to mix it all up before you eat it. And slowly but surely, the other stuff we were so used to eating was on its way out too. Bye-bye potato chips, white bread, sodas, jams and jellies, and all of the other stuff that tasted so good. It was a complete overhaul of how and what we ate, and for the life of me, I just couldn't understand what the big change was all about.

At nine years old, little did I know my mom had it right and did one of the biggest favors she could ever do for me and for our family; she showed us the difference between eating healthy food and eating worthless junk. She knew that the products we were buying from grocery stores and putting into our bodies were not even worthy of being called food. Not only did she know most food was processed and bad, she also knew how bad the sweet foods were for us and how we were all headed for unhealthy times later in life if we kept it up. She knew food labels lied and there were hidden ingredients which were mostly harmful chemicals and other rubbish that was bad for us. She also knew that food companies added unhealthy ingredients to make food last longer and taste better, which in turn was bad news for anyone eating it. Bottom line, she knew we couldn't trust the food industry because, for the most part, they sold lies, not food.

Today, forty years later, the food industry is a much bigger monster, and it's still having its way with us in a very bad way. Oh, it's easy to find good tasting food, but to find real food that's actually good for us to eat is a full-time job. Yes, the food fraud is rampant, and just because you may be buying most or all of your food from the "healthy" and "organic" sections at the grocery store, that doesn't guarantee you're getting truly healthy food either. Although I could easily turn this chapter into a "healthy nutrition" chapter, that's not what this book is about. Instead, I'm going to stay on course and show you how and where the food industry is faking food and feeding us a bunch of garbage just like everyone else in the fitness industry. With this chapter, I'm going to show you exactly how the food industry lies through its labels and hides the truth about the dirty secrets lurking inside its well-thought-out packaging. We'll just see if free-range animals are truly free, if juice is really juice, if the "all natural" labels are "all BS," and just how much the food industry is faking what they're baking.

Labels of Lies

It seems someone is always covering something up in the fitness industry, and food companies and their labels are right there at the top. And boy are they good at it. The FDA and the US Department of Agriculture (USDA) are about as efficient at keeping the food industry regulated as personal training certifications are at keeping bad trainers out of gyms; neither one is doing a good job. And just like the letters signifying a trainer's certifications don't guarantee the training will be good, the writing on most food labels does not guarantee the food will be good—not even close. To help you see through the dirty water that so often dilutes our ability to really see what's in the food we buy, I've made a list called Fake and Bake that will show you the many lies hidden within food and how labels cover up those lies. Take a look, and be prepared to want to grow your own garden and raise your own meat.

Fake and Bake

"Fat Free" – The Big Fat Lie

This is one of the biggest catch-your-eye tricks that food companies use on their labels, and here's exactly how they get away with the big fat lie. The FDA says that if a food has less than 0.5 grams of fat in each serving, then the company can put "Fat Free" on its labels. Even if the entire food package equals only one serving with 0.5 grams of fat in it, it still has 4–5 calories from fat. And what if the food package contains three or four servings? That's 2 grams of fat, which equals 18 calories. According to the FDA, it's still OK for this food to be labeled fat free, which is absolutely not true. Think about trans fat for a minute—the same math I just used goes for this bad boy too. The food package can say "Trans Fat Free" and still have 0.5 grams of trans fat per serving. Pretty slick marketing huh? Here's something else for you to think about: Any time you see "Fat Free" on a label, be very aware; they may have lowered the fat content, but you can bet they replaced it with something just as bad or worse, like more sugar.

"Sugar Free" – A Sweet Trick

With sugar getting a ton of publicity as bad news, along with people trying to cut more sugar from their diets, food companies have had to disguise the sweet stuff by using different names that sound healthy, but they're still sugars. First of all, just like fat free, food companies can put "Sugar Free" on foods with less than 0.5 grams of sugar per serving. We all know now how this can end up as disguised calories when there are multiple servings. As if this wasn't bad enough, there are countless sweeteners disguised on food labels. Some of the more common ones are high fructose corn syrup, evaporated cane juice, brown rice syrup, beet sugar, brown sugar, and anything ending in "ose" like dextrose, fructose, and glucose. Take a good long look at your next food label and see if any of these show up. And then there are the ever-popular sugar alcohols, which are neither sugar nor alcohol, but rather, a very sneaky and dishonest way for food companies to hide sweet calories.

Sugar Alcohols

First of all, sugar alcohols are carbohydrates, but their calorie content is between one-third and one-half of those of all other carbs. So if a food item has 8 grams of sugar alcohol on the label, you can assume that the calorie content of the sugar alcohols is one-half that of all other carbs, or equal to 4 grams instead of 8. Here's the trick: Companies can put as many sugar alcohols in their food as they want and still put "Sugar Free" on their label. Very recently, I had the pleasure of discrediting the "healthy food" claims of a personal trainer who was trying to convince me that he had a really good protein cookie that was of the healthy variety. I had seen these before, but this one, according to him, was the best ever. I asked him to bring one in, and the next day he did. The minute I looked at the label I knew this was about to get bad for him. The "really healthy protein cookie" was as I'd expected, another food item that was camouflaging bad ingredients. For starters, it had the words "Sugar Free," "Protein Packed," "Fat Free," and "Good Source of Fiber" on the packaging—warning number one. Next, the nutritional label said it had zero sugars, but there were 12 grams of sugar alcohols, which equates to around 16–24 calories. The fat content said less than .05 grams, which equals about 4 calories. At this point, there are roughly 20–30 calories per serving not being reported because everything besides the protein is less than .05 grams per serving. Here's the funny part: The cookie was about half the size of a placeholder and it came in a package of six. I asked my friend, "How many people eat just one cookie?" He smiled and said, "I tell most of my clients to eat just two and spread the others out over a few days." I said, "So this 'healthy' cookie is hiding roughly 25 calories for each one, and you said most people you know eat at least two. According to my math, that's 50 extra calories they are unknowingly eating." He said, "There's no way; the calories don't add up." I then explained sugar alcohol calories and the FDA's definition of sugar free and fat free, and he was in absolute shock. Come to find out, he was also a "distributor" of this special cookie so it all makes sense. That was the last time that trainer ever talked to me again about his healthy protein cookie, or any other nutritional topic for that matter. I wonder if he ever told his clients the truth about the cookie; I think you know the answer. Carbohydrates overall can be tricky, and the way food companies deceitfully use their labels to falsely advertise carbs makes them even trickier, just like the "Low Carb" label.

The Low-Carb Lowdown

Low-carbohydrate foods are often labeled with terms like "Net Carbs," Digestible Carbs," and, of course, "Low Carbs." And guess what?

> There is currently no definition from the FDA on what "low carb" actually means, and this opens the door for food companies to lower the boom and cash in on the low-carb craze.

The FDA has, however, sent warning letters to several companies for their "low-carb abuse" and ordered them to make label changes immediately. Here's the trick with low-carb foods in general: Low-carb foods are often highly processed and are made by adding very unhealthy ingredients like hydrogenated oils, lard, sodium, and a little thing called hidden sugars, which we just talked about, to make the food taste better. And just what the heck constitutes a low-carb food anyway? That's just it; the answer is all over the place because different people need different amounts of carbs according to their genetics, activity level, types of activity, body weight, and fitness goals. Food producers could actually do away with low carb labels altogether because they're useless. Just read the nutrition label, and you can determine if a food is low carb enough for you. There are currently many "diets" out there that call for low-carb eating, so watch out when you're buying your supposedly healthy and low-carb foods; they may be low carb, but they're more than likely full of other unhealthy and unidentifiable ingredients. What about "Whole Grain" claims? If a package says "Made with Whole Grains," is it the whole truth?

The "Whole" Truth

Food companies really get their mileage out of the phrase "Made with Whole Grains," but there are two big problems with this. First of all, there's no way of telling how much whole grain is even in the food product. Chances are, most foods advertised as being made with whole grains actually have a very small amount of the whole grain itself with a ton of other very harmful ingredients like sugar and high fructose corn syrup (more sugar) making up the bulk of the food. Take a good look at the ingredient list and not just the protein, carb, and fat breakdown, and you will see the "whole" truth. The second problem with whole grain labels is that whole grains aren't always whole. Many times, the grains have been pulverized into very fine flour. They may contain all the ingredients from the grain, but the resistance to quick digestion is lost, and these grains can spike blood sugars almost just as fast as their refined counterparts (simple sugars). This, as you know, can create quite a problem for someone with diabetes or hypoglycemia (low blood sugar). Since we're on the subject of whole grains, let's talk about the Big G: gluten.

The Gluttony of Gluten

Boy, did the food industry see an opportunity with the huge gluten upheaval and pounce big time! Before I get into it, what the heck is gluten anyway? Gluten is a mixture of two proteins found in wheat, barley, and rye, but is mostly associated with wheat and wheat products. It gives dough and bread that sticky quality and is found in most baked goods. Yes, doughnuts too. Eating gluten does create intestinal and digestive problems for those with celiac disease and those with sensitivities to gluten. However, if neither one of these health issues persists, there's no need to omit gluten from your diet. But the food industry has made such a big deal out of it that it seems everyone should avoid gluten. This is yet another way the food industry is taking advantage of us.

What most people do not know about gluten-free foods is that these foods have been processed. That's right, the very thing every single health resource tells you to avoid: processed foods. So what gives? When foods are stripped of gluten, fiber, vitamins, and minerals are also stripped. And since removing gluten is going to also remove a lot of the taste, highly refined, high-glycemic starches like cornstarch, potato starch, tapioca starch, and sugar are added to the food. This my friend is the very definition of processed food.

In the *ABCnews.go.com* article, "5 Gluten Myths You Were Too Embarrassed to Ask About," author Sydney Lupkin quoted Dr. Kelley Thomsen, gastroenterologist at Vanderbilt University Medical Center, as saying, "There's nothing inherently unhealthy about gluten." The article also explained that "gluten alone doesn't have many health benefits, but foods that contain gluten—like whole grains—tend to be higher in fiber and have a lot of vitamin B, zinc and iron.... As a result, cutting gluten could actually result in nutritional deficiencies."[16]

And to really slap the consumer in the face, most gluten-free foods have higher price tags. How do you feel about gluten-free foods now? At least you know the truth. What about all those fruit juices that claim 100 percent real juice? Can we drink up and not worry, or should we leave it on the shelf?

A Juicy Lie

I know you've seen labels like "100% Real Fruit Juice," "All-Natural Fruit," and "Made from Concentrate," but exactly what do these statements mean and can you trust them? When it comes to fruit and vegetable juices, there are many ways companies can fake it. Let's start with the trickery of the "100% Real Juice" label.

When you see this label, it's easy to assume that you're getting 100 percent real fruit or vegetable juice, right? Here's the truth: Food companies are allowed to put "100% Real Fruit Juice" on the label even though their juice contains additional additives, flavorings, or preservatives. In addition, food companies will dilute their advertised fruit juices with other types of cheaper fruit juices like grape, apple, or pear, all to save money. To sweeten the deal, food companies will also add their number one food additive: SUGAR! You know, just to make sure it tastes good and all. The bottom line is, the juice in the container may well be 100 percent real fruit juice, but real fruit juice may only be 50 percent of what's in the container. To ensure you are definitely getting 100 percent real fruit or vegetable juice, stick to organic or raw juice drinks. Typically, these juices come in clear bottles where you can actually see the fruit or vegetable sediment at the bottom. If the juice is clear and without this sediment, leave it where you found it. And those juice concentrates, watch out for those too.

Juice Concentrate

Have you ever wondered just what in the heck juice concentrate is? I definitely used to. Here you go: Juice concentrate is just another way food companies sabotage us by using shelf-stable juice concentrates instead of real juice. Juice concentrates are made from fruits and vegetables that have been heated to the point where they become syrup. Water is then added back in to bring the volume back up. By the way, heat damages and kills nutrition, so when they heat these juices they're damaging the nutritional content as well. The concentration process also involves both adding and subtracting chemicals and natural plant by-products in order to condense the juice. As you can imagine, the concentration process makes fruits and vegetables lose their flavor, and this is one of the reasons why companies have to re-add "flavoring" to make the juice taste fresh. And the flavoring they add… yep, it's chemical and artificial. The concentration process allows juices to be preserved longer, which in turn allows them to stay on shelves longer and saves the company a ton of money. More lies and more cheap fake food. How about those other "fruit" juices crowding the shelves at the grocery stores—how bad are they?

Fruity Drinks

If I had to pick a mascot for this book, it may well be fruit-flavored drinks because on the outside they look really good and healthy, but on the inside, there's nothing but bad news for your health. Drink companies spend millions of dollars on packaging for these worthless drinks, and they can because the juice inside the package is basically sugar and water. Even though you'll see the phrase "Made with Real/Pure Fruit Juice" on almost all of these cheap fruit drinks, most of them contain only 10 percent or less real fruit juice. And those really sweet fruit flavorings that kids love are chemicals and artificial flavorings. Remember, all a company has to do to justify the words "Made with Real Fruit" on their label is to have just a tiny bit of real fruit in the drink. Period! That's it!

Now that you've seen how food companies use fake and bake cover-ups for their cheap foods and drinks, I want to show you a much broader and bolder way they lure us into their tasteless traps. I'm talking about labels that have nothing to do with taste, but rather, labels about how the company's food is grown or raised. Do these labels have any credibility, or are they deceitful and untrustworthy like all the other labels we just talked about? I'll let you make that decision. Take a look at my Tasteless Traps list and see if any of these leave a bad taste in your mouth.

Tasteless Traps

All-Natural Liar

In addition to the FDA regulating most of our food, we have the USDA, which regulates meat and poultry, but they basically do the same things. And when it comes to the phrase "All Natural" we see on food labels, including meat, fish, and poultry, neither the FDA nor the USDA has an official definition of the term "natural" or its derivatives. They only go so far as to say they don't object to the use of the term "if the food does not contain added color, artificial flavors, or synthetic substances," which gives companies pretty generous leeway. Basically, food companies can put whatever they want into food and call it all natural and get away with feeding us yet another plate full of you know what.

In my opinion, there are two huge problems with the label "All Natural." First, the ingredients in most foods with this label are anything but natural; they're chemicals, preservatives, artificial colors, dyes, and flavors, and countless other things we can't even pronounce. Here's a rule of thumb when it comes to ingredients in any food item: If you can't make the food in your own kitchen, and if you can't pronounce or define all of the ingredients on the label, it's not natural, and it will do unnatural things inside your body. Second, even though a food may actually be all natural, it doesn't mean it's good for you. Some foods are naturally high in cholesterol and other fats, sugar, and sodium, making them foods to either eat on occasion in small amounts, or to avoid altogether. There are all-natural ice creams, doughnuts, bacon and other meats, dressings, candy, and many other foods that can wreck your health if you eat too much of them. Believe me, if I could live off ice cream and be healthy, I'd do it. The bottom line is not to trust a label that says "All Natural" because chances are that label is there to cover up something the food company doesn't want you to see. What about the new go-to term, "artisan," which seems to be everywhere? Is this just another ploy food companies use to sell their fake food as something natural and healthy?

A Lost Art

The "Artisan" label evokes images of small-batch cooking and skilled chefs who shopped farmer's markets and local gardens for fresh ingredients. But it's a word not regulated by the FDA, which means anyone can use it any way they want—even with bulk quantities of frozen foods, breads, fast foods, pizzas, and just about any other foods for that matter. Here's what artisan really means, according to *Dictionary.com*: *A person skilled in an applied art, or a person or company that makes a high-quality and distinctive product in small quantities, usually by hand or by using traditional methods.*

Basically, artisan food is made by hand, from scratch, with truly all-natural, organic ingredients, and in small quantities. Now, does that sound like a food you would get from a drive-up window at a fast-food joint? Or do you think there is a group of chefs in those tall white hats behind the frozen food section at your grocery store who are making all of those artisan frozen foods and pizzas by hand? Exactly! Don't be fooled by this new go-to label trick by food companies; it's still nothing but trash. And watch out for the "Organic" label; there are tricks-a-plenty with this one too.

Farm Fresh or Barnyard BS?

This is actually the one place where we can feel pretty good about the food we eat, but you still have to be careful. "Organic" is a powerful word in the food and diet industry, and just like all other food lies, it can be misleading. But there are ways to know for sure whether your food is farm fresh or whether it's nothing more than barnyard BS. The USDA and the FDA have some pretty clear definitions of what organic really means, but there are different levels at which a food can be determined as truly organic. Let's start with 100 percent organic and work our way down.

100% Organic

Products labeled "100% Organic" and carrying the "USDA Organic" seal adhere to strict, legal standards and must be verified as meeting the specific requirements of "organic" by a USDA-accredited certifying agent. If a company is caught knowingly selling or mislabeling their goods as organic, or the product was not produced and handled in accordance with the USDA regulations, the company can be subject to a civil penalty of up to $10,000 per violation. Furthermore, organic meat, poultry, eggs, and dairy products are required to come from animals that are given no anti-biotics or growth hormones. Organic food is produced without using most conventional pesticides; fertilizers made with synthetic ingredients or sewage sludge; bioengineering; or ionizing radiation. How does "sewage sludge" sit with you? Pretty dang nasty, isn't it? But it does show up in many of our foods. Next up, just plain old "organic."

Organic

The difference between 100 percent organic and just organic is that organic products have to be 95 percent organic instead of 100 percent. Usually, these are pretty safe, and you can quickly check the ingredient label to see what that other 5 percent may be. Chances are, it's OK, but check just to be safe. In order for any food to be declared as truly organic, it must not have any of these ingredients or processes:

- Antibiotics

- Artificial growth hormones

- High fructose corn syrup

- Artificial dyes (made from coal tar and petrochemicals)

- Artificial sweeteners derived from chemicals

- Synthetically created chemical pesticide and fertilizers

- Genetically engineered proteins and ingredients

- Sewage sludge – NASTY!

- Irradiation

You do know where this list comes from, right? These are the very things that are commonly found in a lot of our foods, including the ones that claim to be all natural. Have you started tilling the soil for your new garden and building your own chicken coup yet? It's pretty scary, isn't it? As you can see, eating organic is your safest bet in terms of getting real food, but there's another level of organic where you have to keep one eye open.

Made with Organic Ingredients

Foods with this labeling must consist of at least 70 percent organic ingredients, and none of the ingredients can be produced with sewage-sludge-based products or ionizing radiation. Labeling cannot include the USDA seal or the word "organic" in any principal displays. Three of the organic ingredients can be included on the label, but the label cannot use "organic" as a stand-alone word. All organic ingredients should be identified in the ingredients list, and the same controls and regulations are put in place as those used for foods labeled organic. There are strict restrictions on the other 30 percent of ingredients, and these cannot have any genetically modified organisms.

As you can see, organic is a good thing as long as it fits the above criteria. And yes, you'll pay more for truly organic foods because of the higher costs of growing or raising these foods, but when it comes to not poisoning your body with all the other BS that goes into our food, the price is right! What about the other labels food companies use that aren't so much about taste as they are about quality, like "Free Range/Cage Free"? Are these misleading and abused phrases as well?

Home on the Range

The first thing to know about labels that claim "Free Range" or "Cage Free" is that these labels are very minimally regulated. Here's the trick: Although the USDA says that to put these terms on labels the animals cannot be contained in any way and must be allowed to roam and forage freely over a large area of open land, food companies easily get away with not abiding by these specifications. The very definition of this regulation has more holes than a field of groundhogs. The words "roam," "forage," and "large area of open land" all are open to a wide array of interpretations, and companies have a field day with it—pun intended. If called upon by the USDA, all a food producer has to do is demonstrate that the animals are allowed access to "large open areas."

The USDA explains Free Range or Free Roaming as, "Producers must demonstrate to the agency that the poultry has been allowed access to the outside."[17] Just because they have "access" to these large areas for grazing and running doesn't mean they get to do it a lot or at all. And there are no definitions of "large open areas" and "free to roam," so let the games begin. Here's another huge void in this regulation: Food producers do not have to apply or become certified to put "Free Range" or "Cage Free" on their food labels. They can put it on all of their food products without proving it. How's that for trustworthy regulations? And then there's the whole "Grass Fed" label; are animals really being fed grass or something else we don't know about?

The Graze Craze

Does the label "Grass Fed" on meat packaging carry any merit at all? It's really hard to tell because as with free range and cage free, there is very minimal regulation from the USDA. The first problem with trusting this label is that just because an animal is grass fed doesn't mean it hasn't been contained and packed in with many other animals. And even though the labels "Free Range" and "Cage Free" might accompany the "Grass Fed" label, this doesn't guarantee anything, as you saw in the previous paragraph. So if you ever see "Grass Fed and Cage Free" on a tofurkey label, this should be a dead giveaway that something is a little off. The second problem is the lack of proof and regulation by the USDA to assure us that the meat or poultry we are getting was indeed from 100 percent grass-fed animals. And the last problem, most grass-fed animals tend to weigh less and gain weight slower than grain-fed animals, so what do some food producers do? They turn their animals over to grain feeding during the last months of their lives so they gain weight before they are slaughtered and processed. Some grass-fed claims are legit, but you really have to know your meat source to fully verify this. The only true way is to know exactly where your meat comes from and actually see for yourself how the animals are being raised. But watch out, you might just step in something that stinks. Or you could just eat at healthy fast-food places.

Fast-Food Fallacy

To keep up with the times, most fast-food restaurants are getting in on the health-food kick by adding "healthy" items to their menus, adding "artisan" foods, and even being so brave as to list the nutritional values for their food items. Here's what you need to know about "healthy fast food" and it's really simple: ALL fast food is cheap, not only in price but in quality as well. How in the world do you think they make money by selling hamburgers and tacos for under four dollars? They buy very low-grade and low-quality food from their vendors, cook it in very cheap ways, and slide it under the heat lamp where it waits for its lucky and hungry new owner to "drive up to the second window please." Over the years, I've had numerous clients tell me they're eating healthy, only to discover they have been frequenting fast-food places. And after I bust them they always say things like, "I only ate half the bun," "I got a salad with chicken," "It was off their healthy menu," and "I didn't eat the fries." And again, I remind them that when they eat at fast-food places, they aren't eating food, they're eating poison in the form of chemical sludge and cardboard disguised as meat. And that weight they didn't lose, which they have been working so hard to lose—those umpteen million grams of sodium didn't help one bit with that either.

Bottom line: There is no such thing as healthy fast food, period!

No matter what that new "health conscious" menu says. So far, most of these tasteless traps have been about meat and dairy products, but what about those labels claiming vegan ingredients? Are they all 100 percent free of animal products?

Vegan Victims

It's hard enough to find clean, wholesome foods to eat, but when it comes to finding foods that are truly vegan, that's an even bigger challenge. As with all other foods, it's easy for the food industry to put a misleading vegan label on foods that end up having meat products in the ingredients, so I've got a few ways for you vegans out there to make sure you're truly getting 100 percent plant-based products.

The first thing you can do is **check for cholesterol.** If the product has any cholesterol at all, even just 1 milligram, this means there is some sort of animal-derived ingredient present in the food. However, at the same time, if it has no cholesterol, it doesn't automatically qualify the food as truly vegan. The next thing you can check is the **allergy listing** on the food package. Most, if not all, foods have at the end of their ingredient list a list of common allergens, which includes milk, egg, soy, and wheat. Sometimes the common allergens are printed in boldface in the ingredient list to make them stand out. If the list has anything non-vegan, go ahead and put it back on the shelf. And last, **look for animal-derived ingredients.** There are several, but these are the most common ones: vitamin D3 (rarely vegan, but D2 always is), whey, honey, lactose, and casein (a milk protein that sometimes finds its way into things like soy cheese). Be wary of items with "natural flavors," but "artificial flavors" shouldn't be an issue, unless you're trying to avoid those for different reasons. Eating healthy is definitely a challenge, but eating vegan takes a much sterner studying of ingredients and their sources of processing. Before I close this section, there are a few other Tasteless Traps I want to mention, and although these are not along the same lines as the others we've talked about so far, they are indeed traps.

Getting Served

One of the big things I have to continually point out to my clients is to be very aware of serving sizes and the number of servings in the foods they eat. It's easy to look at a food label and see the total calories, fat, sugar, and carbohydrates, but a good look into the serving size and how many servings are in the package is largely neglected—or intentionally ignored. One very good trick food companies play on us is putting phrases like "1/3 fewer calories," "1/3 less sodium," and "1/3 less fat," on their labels. But what they don't tell you is they more than likely lowered the serving size and kept the calories, sodium, fat, and everything else the same. I told you this was a good trick! And the other part of the calorie trap is not looking at the number of servings. The number of servings of some foods can get way up there with candy and most junk food, but it can happen on any food package. When you look at a food label, be sure to look at the serving size, and then multiply the total calories by the number of servings to get the total caloric and other nutrient amounts in the whole package of food. The best example of this is with candy and potato chips. Take a look at the label on one of these foods the next time you're in the grocery store and see how many servings are in each package. I hate to say this because I love it like crazy, but chocolate is one of the worst in terms of the number of servings in a very small package. Don't be mad at me! I know we've talked about ingredients a lot so far, but there's one more thing you need to know about them, and it's a big one.

First on the List

When you look at the ingredient list on a food package, just know that the ingredients are listed in order from the most common to the least common. This will help you determine just how much of the advertised ingredient is actually in the food. Ideally, you want the ingredient list to be very short with nothing but the actual food itself, but if there are a few other ingredients, make sure the one you're buying is the very first on the list. Believe it or not, there are many foods where the second ingredient is only 1 percent of the product and then the following ingredient amounts decline from there. Read those labels guys! Food, which is truly organic, will almost always just have the food itself listed in the ingredients and nothing else.

Eating clean is a full-time job, but once you know how to spot the dirty truths hiding throughout the food industry, your path to healthier eating won't be so rough. From "Sugar Free" and "All Natural," to "Low Fat" and "Gluten Free," the labels of lies will lure you in and make you feel good about your food choices. But it's all one big food fight with fraud coming out on top, leaving you with nothing but a bag-o-fakeness. To avoid the food scam, you have to keep your eyes peeled and read between, under, on top, and behind the lines of ingredients to spot the fake and bake ways of food companies because they do the exact same things that the rest of the fitness industry does.

They disguise cheap, fake, and over-promising products with pretty packages and hope nobody knows the difference.

But they're not the only ones selling food fraud as a package deal. There's another industry making millions with their "losing" ways.

9 The Skinny on Weight-Loss Plans and Scams

Have you ever played the dice game craps? Whew, now that's a hell of an exciting game. You've got a table full of hyped up, adrenalin-fueled thrill seekers all hoping for the exact same thing: that the dice keep landing on the good numbers. And you can always tell when a table gets hot; everyone is screaming, slapping high fives, and smiling from ear to ear because they're making money and having a blast doing it. And on the other side of the coin, you can definitely tell which tables are cold as ice because it's quiet, nobody is smiling, and people are starting to walk away because they're losing their a**es. The game of craps offers countless ways to win, and when you see how the table is laid out with all the big and bright numbers, it makes you feel that this game is a sure bet. Add the excitement, thrill, and adrenalin-filled anticipation of becoming a big winner, and people line up to throw their money down. But the truth is, as exciting and enticing as craps is, it will take your money and take it fast, leaving you feeling let down and wondering, "What the hell just happened?"

> In truth, shooting dice is a lot like taking your chances
> with weight-loss companies and fad diets: There's a lot
> of excitement, which draws you in; you're with a lot of
> people all wanting the same outcome; it looks like the
> odds are in your favor; and the house makes all its
> money off losers.

Weight-loss companies lure people in with "losing weight is easy" campaigns, emotional testimonials, and celebrity endorsements, but many leave their customers losing a lot more than weight. Whether it's a ridiculous "20 pounds in 10 days" fad diet plan, or a more respectable and gradual weight-loss program that offers account-ability and support, all weight-loss programs have skeletons in their closets. In his blog, "4 Top Weight Loss Scams of the Year (So Far)," author William Anderson wrote of deceptive marketing and false advertising charges that the Federal Trade Commission brought against four weight-loss companies. "However, don't expect this to stop them," he wrote. "The FTC has been catching these frauds for years. They just pop back up the next year with new gimmicks with new names and sales pitches."[18]

In this chapter, I'm going to show you how really whacky fad diets are and how they leave you much worse off than when you started. And all of those well-known national weight-loss companies—I'll show you exactly where some of these companies are causing you to lose much more than your weight. What about the never-ending merry-go-round of opinions on what's really healthy to eat and what's not? In this chapter, you'll learn how to tell if you're really getting good advice or if you're being fed a bunch of bologna.

Let's get started by taking a closer look into where crash diets and weight-loss plans are going wrong and causing their customers to end up on the losing end of weight loss.

The Losing End of Weight Loss

The Fad is Bad!

Just as multi-level marketing companies prey on their prospect's hopes and dreams of a better financial future, many fad diet and weight-loss plans prey on people's enduring desires to lose weight and feel good about the way they look. And when someone who has battled weight gain for a large part of their life hears a "you can lose 20 pounds in 10 days" pitch, they're all ears. I don't blame people at all for falling for these quick and drastic weight-loss fads, but at the same time, I want to expose these whacko diet plans for what they really are and lead people to much healthier ways of weight loss. Losing weight this fast is not good, and in most cases, it's very harmful and can lead to serious health issues. Take a look at all the ways fad diets are bad for you, and hopefully you'll see why these diets leave people worse off than before they started them.

Short-Term Loss

Yes, it's true you might lose ten pounds in two weeks, but you'll probably gain twenty pounds in one month after you stop the faddy crash diet. These diets aren't designed for long-term loss because the extremely calorie-restrictive methods cannot be sustained from both a physical and emotional standpoint. And as soon as you come off these types of diets, you'll more than likely go back to eating like you did before, and the weight you lost will find you soon, and then some. I'm going to make this really simple: Any diet plan that advertises super-quick weight loss is no good. The companies that sell these plans are only in it for your money, and they know exactly what to say to get you to buy into their magic weight-be-gone plans, so don't waste your health, your money, or your water on these no-good plans. That's right, I said water.

"Waisting" Water

Any time quick weight loss happens, it's almost always just water. Why is this? It's very simple. One of the signature methods of quick weight-loss diets is to greatly restrict your carbohydrate intake. When you eat carbohydrates, your body breaks them down and stores them as glucose in your blood and as glycogen in your liver and muscles. Here's the catch: With every gram of glycogen you store, there will be 2–3 grams of water stored as well. So when a diet calls for carbohydrate restriction, your body loses its glycogen stores and the water stored with it. Therefore, most—if not all—of those ten pounds you lost in two weeks were just water. And those inches they promised you'd lose off your waist... yep, that was water too. So not only are you not losing body fat, you're losing water, electrolytes, and other nutrients, which can all lead to dehydration and a severe strain on your organs. Unfortunately, water isn't the only loss you'll have.

The Real Loss

Foolish fad diets are harmful and worthless; this is the only way to say it. What they promise and what you'll actually get are two completely different things. In addition to losing crucial water and electrolytes, other bodily functions like hormone production, energy, and maintaining muscle mass all take a direct hit. These crazy diets greatly restrict your calories, causing your entire body to slow down and run at a much less efficient rate. When this happens, your metabolism slows down (the very thing you want to increase), your energy drops, and your body will actually start burning muscle for energy. These are all very negative things and can affect you for the rest of your life. Muscle is gold when it comes to metabolism, and if you lose it your metabolism will drop, and your losses will begin to mount against you. Fad diets do absolutely nothing to benefit you because they're so short lived, they fake real weight loss as water, and they cause you to end up worse off than when you began, over and over again. So are there any weight-loss plans that are good and truly help people lose body fat? Yes, they are out there, but you have to do your research. Always take a close look at a plan to see where it might lead you astray, and be prepared to hit the brakes.

Getting the Skinny

Before you go "all in" and invest your hopes in one of the countless weight-loss plans blasted all over TV and social media promising a smaller, thinner, happier, and more productive you, slow down and take a real close look at exactly what it is they're offering to help you lose. Weight-loss companies have figured out the perfect formula to get your attention and your money: They catch your eyes and ears with a celebrity endorsement, share emotional weight-loss struggles and successes of "satisfied product users," and tell you just how easy it really is to get your high school body back. I know in the previous chapters I already covered how fitness advertisements mislead consumers by playing on their emotions and using pre-fit models to advertise their goods, but I'm going to give you more specific things to watch out for when it comes to weight-loss plans and their "skinny can be yours" offers. I actually do think there are some pretty good plans out there that provide accountability and overall good guidance, but even with the top-tiered weight-loss plans, there are several things you should know before you "Order Now!" Here is my list of Weight Loss Whoas, reminding you to pump those brakes before you get waist deep in any weight-loss plan.

Weight Loss Whoas – Hitting the Brakes!

Do Your Homework

Doing your research and getting unbiased ratings and testimonials about weight-loss plans and companies is the most valuable thing you can do before you buy into any of these programs. Be careful of your search results because many of these companies do their own reviews and post them under different articles that seem to be unbiased, so be sure you use reliable sources. Major TV networks do these kinds of reviews often, and you can also use sources like WebMD, the American Heart Association, the Mayo Clinic, and other national health organizations. Remember, fraud runs deep in the fitness industry, and weight-loss companies are definitely not immune to it. Once you have done your research, you can take a good look at exactly what it is they want you to eat or drink.

Food Monopoly

Watch out for this one! Some weight-loss companies make it mandatory or pressure people into using their food only, and even though their food may be OK and healthy, it still limits your ability to eat healthy. And just because they're selling the food doesn't guarantee that it's of good quality. You've got a whole chapter on how the food industry lies and fakes food, so if you do buy your food from weight-loss companies, ask them where their food comes from, if it's truly organic, and how it is they get their information about their food. In my opinion, people should be taught to both buy and prepare healthy foods on their own with an option to purchase food from the plan itself. Companies may say they are doing this out of convenience but I don't buy it; I feel they are just using this to create more income for the company. Either way you look at it, people should be able to both buy food from the company itself and buy and prepare their own food when it comes to losing weight. Most of these companies preach that losing weight is a lifestyle change; being forced to buy pre-made food doesn't constitute a "lifestyle change" in my book. And those "certified" nutritionists and other weight-loss "professionals" that companies supposedly have on staff—are they really qualified to teach you anything?

Disqualified Experts

Just as personal trainers have worthless certifications, there are plenty of "nutrition experts" who have worthless credentials working within many weight-loss companies. Many of these companies will say they have licensed dieticians and certified nutritionists drawing up their meal plans, but how do we know this is true?

We don't! In addition to asking companies about the sources of their "healthy" foods, ask them about the people designing their meal plans as well. And their so-called nutrition advisers—how much experience do you think they actually have in prescribing diets? These are questions you should ask before signing up for any weight-loss plan. And don't let them get by with vague or redirecting questions; make them tell you the truth. Better yet, take this book with you and let the questioning begin. What about weight-loss plans that include supplements? Is this a big red light?

Supplemental Income

I'll keep this short because we've already covered how most supplements are bogus, but with some weight-loss plans, supplements play a big part. I will tell you to be very leery of a weight-loss plan that requires and pushes the use of supplements. In addition to having the big problem of many supplements not being of good quality, we have the problem of supplements being unnecessary. Even though I think there are certain vitamin and mineral supplements that are necessary, most supplement use is overkill. If a weight-loss plan is adding supplements to your diet, make the company tell you why. Ask them why their diet needs supplementation if it is indeed "healthy" and adequate. Also ask them exactly who is making their supplements, and be on the lookout for those proprietary blends. Watch out for supplement sales in any form, ask a lot of questions, and do your research. And above all, if a weight-loss plan claims some sort of "magic weight-loss pill" as a "big part of their success," don't even consider this plan as an option; you already know why. What about those plans that say, "No Exercise Needed"? Does this mean the plan is super-duper good, or is this a sign telling you to drop this plan and run?

The Exercise Exit

This one makes me laugh. Look, it's pretty straightforward: Any plan that says you don't have to exercise is BS. "No Exercise Required" is a very popular statement made by many fad and other diet plans, and because I've heard it hundreds of times, I can just about recite the irrational sales pitch that goes with it: "Are you tired of spending countless hours at the gym, walking during your lunch hour, or doing one of those crazy exercise videos and not losing a pound? Don't worry; those days are over! All you have to do is follow our professionally guided nutrition plan, drink our scientifically formulated weight-loss and energy drink twice a day, and you'll lose weight without ever exercising again. That's right! You'll eat delicious and nutritious foods made by our gourmet chefs from all-natural ingredients. You'll even get to eat dessert twice a day and still lose weight! Exercise? No way! All you have to do is start following our new weight-be-gone plan and the weight will instantly start to fall off." It sounds silly, doesn't it? But this is exactly how they sound. The bottom line: Steer clear of any program that tells you no exercise is needed; they couldn't care less if you're healthy or not.

Getting the skinny on a weight-loss plan before you sign up can make the biggest difference of all in whether you're losing weight in a healthy way or just losing water and money. Don't just take the company's word for how on-the-level they are; do your research, ask many questions, and don't let them skimp on their answers. And if they can't answer your questions in specific and rational ways, write them off and move on.

As you can see, the food industry from top to bottom is questionable, and there is nothing about it in which we can fully trust. Even when everyone agrees exactly what healthy food really is, all of a sudden there's a 180-degree turn, and the food that was healthy yesterday is bad and causes all kinds of health problems today. One day fat and carbs are good and the next day they're nuclear waste. And those food labels we talked about earlier—companies play right along and change the words as needed to reflect the current idea of what is and isn't healthy. Throw in the millions of "nutrition experts" with their opinions on what's good and bad and you have the perfect recipe for confusion and frustration when it comes to knowing what the heck is truly healthy to eat. There's only one true way to end the confusion and get peace of mind that your way of eating is healthy: You have to quit relying on everybody else and learn for yourself.

Opinions on healthy eating are a lot like Texas weather: If you don't like what it currently is, just hang on because it's going to change in an instant. From "low fat" and "low carb," to "don't eat meat" and "egg yolks are bad," opinions on how to truly eat healthy are contradictory, confusing, and short lived. Even though there are some things that almost everyone agrees are healthy for us to eat, there are foods that constantly go back and forth on the good versus bad list. This is because of two main reasons: First, it's because scientists in a laboratory somewhere gave mice an extremely unnatural amount of a certain food over and over again, which caused the mice to have health problems or die. And second, some individual or group who typically has an alternative agenda uses factually challenged and emotional propaganda to scare people into eating a certain way. The news spreads, people panic, and the big swap from meat to veggies or from carbs to fat happens almost overnight. And then look out! It's all over the news that a certain food is all of a sudden bad for us to eat. Let's cut to the chase here. The only way to avoid confusion, bias, and bad nutritional advice is to educate yourself on the macronutrients (carbs, proteins, and fats) and how your body uses them in different ways. My next list, Clean Your Plate, will help you determine for yourself just how much good or bad food ends up on your fork or spoon.

Clean Your Plate

Carbs Get a Bad Rap

This is probably the most confusing part of healthy eating across the board because of pure ignorance and misunderstanding of what carbohydrates really do. Carbohydrates are the key to any diet because they are the most efficient and easily attainable energy source for your body; you just have to monitor the type, the amount, and the timing of when you eat them. But there are uninformed and uneducated people claiming carbs are the enemy, and they couldn't be more wrong. I hear people all the time say, "I've cut out all of my carbs," and "I'm not eating any sugars," and I just have to laugh because that's impossible to do and still be healthy. First of all, all carbs are sugars; some are simple sugars (sweeteners, fruits, sugar), and some are complex sugars (wheat, rice, potatoes, nuts, pasta, quinoa, bread, whole grains, and vegetables). When people say they have cut out all sugars, they are typically referring to the simple sugars like candy, sweeteners, and sodas. And when they say they are cutting out all carbs, they mean they have cut out wheat products, rice, pasta, potatoes, breads, etc. And what about fruit? Fruit is a simple carbohydrate that contains fiber (a complex carb that has no nutritional value), but it's still a sugar, so you can easily see how this whole carb thing gets completely off track. Here's a little something to help you get started in understanding carbohydrates.

Without getting my lab coat and beakers out, simple carbs are broken down and enter into your blood quickly (within ten or twenty minutes), and complex carbs are broken down and enter into your blood over a longer period of time (one and a half to two hours). To start learning how fast or slowly different carbs enter your blood, you can look for a glycemic index on the labels of packaged foods, or you can look up an online glycemic index, which will list common foods and how quickly the carbs enter your blood. This is where the type, the amount, and the timing of your carbohydrate intake comes into play.

> If you get this right for your genetics, activity level, and body weight goals, carbs will be your new best friend— not the enemy so many uninformed people claim.

The Protein Shake-Up

I have a very good friend who used to work out with me a few years back, and he was always drinking something when he arrived for our workouts. One day I finally asked him, "What's in the drink?" He said, "Protein. What else would it be, stupid?" I said, "So, you're already done working out?" He said, "No, dummy; we're just about to start. Why are you asking?" I then told him that all that protein he was drinking wasn't going to do him much good at that point and that it may even slow him down during his workouts because it's going to just sit in his stomach. I explained to him that his pre-workout food should be mostly complex carbohydrates consumed one and a half to two hours before a workout so that the nutrition can be digested, processed, and stored as energy. I also told him that his protein drink should be consumed after his workout to start repairing and recuperating his body. He was mad because I waited so long to tell him, but I thought he was drinking an energy drink or water instead of protein. He made the switch and guess what happened to his workouts? They improved across the board, and he wasn't mad anymore.

Protein is not a good source of energy, plain and simple. It is a source of energy if you make your body use it but it comes with a price. Protein's main job in the human body is to support blood, muscle, bone, and hormone production—not energy as many people think. When your body is made to use protein as energy because of carbohydrate and fat restriction, your blood, muscles, bones, and hormones lose out because you're using up protein for energy. This is what I mean by the timing of your macronutrients (carbs, proteins, and fats); if you eat the right amounts at the right times, your body will operate on a very efficient level. Like I said previously, avoid having a protein drink before you work out, have a small amount of protein, a small amount of fat, and mostly complex carbs one and a half to two hours prior to your workout instead. After your workout, eat mostly protein, a moderate amount of complex carbs, and a moderate amount of fat. The exact percentages of macronutrients vary from one person to another, but remember, protein is for recuperation, not energy. So far, we've talked about carbohydrates and protein; what's left? Good old fat!

No Fat—No Chance

One of the biggest mistakes people make when trying to eat healthier and lose weight is cutting too much fat from their diets. I'm all for eliminating trans fats and greatly limiting the amount of LDL cholesterol (the bad kind), but other than that, we need fat as a staple in our diets to function in healthy ways. This is an area you're going to need to spend a little time researching, but I'll give you a good start. For most people, a diet should consist of about 20–25 percent fat calories. Some people go down to 15 percent and some up to 30 percent, but it depends on the variables I've mentioned before: body type, activity level, activity type, body weight, and overall fitness goals. In addition, roughly 7–10 percent of a person's total daily calories should be from saturated fats. That's right, although we have to greatly limit our saturated fat intake, we still need it to be healthy. Did you know that saturated fat is a healthy component in every cell in our bodies? Our cell membranes are made up of cholesterol (saturated fat), and if there isn't enough saturated fat, our cells become less healthy. And that little thing called mitochondria inside our cells—it takes a big hit too. Use resources like the Mayo Clinic, WebMD, and the American Heart Association to learn about good versus bad fats and exactly how much may be right for you.

Trying your luck with weight-loss companies is definitely a crapshoot; some will get you excited when good numbers show up, and some will turn ice cold, take your money, and leave you thinking, "WTH?" To avoid burning money with nothing to show, avoid the "lose weight fast" plans and while you're at it, be sure you get the real skinny by researching the company and their weight-loss ways so that you don't end up on the losing end of everything but your weight. Last, do yourself a favor and become nutritionally independent by cleaning your plate of all the confusing, misleading, and constantly changing opinions on exactly what's healthy to eat by learning about food for yourself. Do these things, and you'll end up on the winning side of the losing industry.

The US government tells us we need to eat healthier and make better food choices, yet they are the ones skimping on the quality control side of things. But why break precedence? The government and the food industry seem like they're just following the lead of everyone else in the fitness industry where fakeness is natural and true health has taken a backseat. As I said in my introduction to this book, the fitness industry is out of shape, and if big changes aren't made very soon, the very heart of fitness, which is supposed to be pure, clean, and natural will forever be tainted and fake. And true health will be a thing of the past.

10 Breaking Bad: Fixing a Broken Industry

Between the ages of seven and thirteen I spent my summers busting my butt working for my dad in one of the hottest and dirtiest occupations on the planet: the oil patch. It was during these hot and seemingly never-ending days when my dad used grit, relentless hard work, and tough love to pound some of life's toughest lessons into my young mind. With my dad, it was all about hard work, respect, and character, and if I ever crossed the line, I paid the price, right then and right there. I'll never forget the day two other boys and I were given the job of painting pumpjacks. In case you don't know, pumpjacks are those things that go up and down and pump oil out of the ground, and they are filthy, covered in more grease and dirt than you could ever imagine. The first thing we had to do was use screwdrivers and putty knives to scrape off inches of packed-on grease and dirt that had accumulated over the years. Second, we had to use gasoline and wire brushes to scrub the pumpjacks down to the metal. Last, we had to paint them with two coats of bright blue paint. After doing this routine on three or four of these things in one-hundred-degree heat, it got old really quick. So we decided we would "speed up the process" by skipping a few steps. I mean, who's really going to notice anyway, being way out in the country and everything? On our fifth pumpjack, we skipped the degreasing and gasoline scrub and went straight to painting, right on top of all the grease. We all stood back, took a good look, and decided it looked as good as all the others. So what did we do? We did the same thing to the next units until our day was done.

The next day we were driving up to start working on the remaining pumpjacks, and there stood my dad by one of the units we had painted the day before. As we walked up, you could see these huge globs of blue grease on the ground where they had fallen off the pumpjack, and I knew my a** was in for it. My dad simply told the other two boys to go back to the shop to work there for the day, and after they left my dad looked at me and said, "You should have known better, son. I don't care whose idea it was, it was your responsibility to do the job right. You took the cheap way out, you did a poor job, and you lied to me. Now it's on you to make it right."

I had to completely redo the pumpjacks we had already painted and finish the rest of them all by myself, fourteen in total. It took me a whole week of twelve-hour days to finish that job, and on the very night I finished, I was lying in bed about to go to sleep when my dad came into my room and said, "Son, I'm proud of you; you did a great job. Now get some sleep." I was feeling pretty good until what he said next. He said, "I've been thinking about it, and I think those pumpjacks would look even better painted black instead of blue; you can start tomorrow."

That was a heck of a tough lesson to learn and one that I thought was going to kill me before I was done, but it didn't. The funny thing is, the lesson really didn't have anything to do with hard work; it was about always having integrity, character, and honesty, especially when nobody is watching you. I learned that whether you get caught at cheating or not isn't the issue; the fact is, if you cheat, you cheat yourself and everyone else involved, and that's the biggest matter of all. I've held tight to that lesson since that day, and when it comes to people trusting me by putting their health in my hands over my nearly three decades in this business, it's the most important lesson I've ever learned.

While its job is to teach, provide, and promote health and longevity, the health and fitness industry is instead providing unlimited opportunities for cheats, scams, and ridiculously fraudulent activity—all to take advantage of the hopes and dreams of millions who want to live longer and healthier lives.

> From fitness instructors and fitness competitors; to
> advertisements, supplements, and the food industry;
> millions of individuals and companies are cheating,
> taking short cuts, and covering up a bunch of dirty lies
> and a lesson on integrity and character is long overdue.

It's time to break the bad out of this industry and send the carnival acts packing, and phony fitness instructors and their circus acts should lead the way.

When it comes to fitness instructors and their methods of exercise, it's a wide-open total body free-for-all to do whatever the heck they want. They certainly know how to bring the pain, count to fifteen, and check their phones; and a lot of them are really good at playing doctor and diagnosing injuries too. But as far as really knowing safe, effective, and productive exercise principles and methods, most of them are better suited supervising a bounce house for kids. To rid the industry of these cartilage killers, we need to start by putting them on the spot. If you currently have a trainer, attend an exercise class at the gym, or partake in a boot camp, see how much your instructor sweats when you ask them specific questions about the way they're having you exercise, and don't accept simple answers. Throw in some specific muscle questions, and if you're having pain during and after your workout, ask them why it's OK to exercise with pain. Above all, if your instructor can't answer your questions with very specific and rational answers, if they sit down while you're training, if they look at their phones during your session, if they tell you they can fix your pain, and if they make you work through any kind of joint or muscle pain, they are idiots and you need to walk away while you can. The truth is, there just aren't many good instructors out there, and whether they're certified or not has absolutely nothing to do with it.

For the most part, fitness instructor certifications might as well be hidden at the bottom of cereal boxes; they're just not that valuable. Those letters look good next to a name, but with the exception of very few certifications, those letters mean only that someone gave a credit card number, took an open-book test, and presto; they officially became a certified fitness instructor. Anyone and everyone can be a fitness instructor, and that's a big problem.

So how do we fix it? The first thing we need to do is require everyone seeking a fitness instructor certification to complete a physical therapy internship of at least six months before taking a certification course. Second, the applicant needs to stand in front of a panel of orthopedic surgeons and physical therapists and answer questions about their training methods and how to deal with injuries; this will weed out most of them. Last, instead of worthless CECs every two years, all fitness instructors should have to demonstrate their training methods in front of another panel of orthopedic surgeons and PTs and be ready to answer questions; this one will definitely send many fitness instructor wannabes looking for another line of work. Incompetent fitness instructors are bad enough, but when you add the immense flex appeal of an industry filled with drug-fit bodies, the entire show takes a very bad turn.

> As a nation and as individuals, is it our true goal to be healthier or to just look healthier with the use of testosterone and other fitness drugs?

The answer is obvious. From professional bodybuilders and fitness competitors, to the sixty-year-old walking around with a twenty-year-old body, drugs are as common as protein powders and yoga pants. And as many people trade in their health card for a needle full of quick-fit and fat-be-gone, they lie and say their new fit look is from nothing other than exercise and eating right, leaving many uninformed people disappointed and wondering why they can't look like that too. Drug use in the fitness industry and the lies that go with it have completely diluted what fit and healthy should really look like, and as you saw from Chapters 3 and 4, it's much more widespread than most people know.

There are only two ways to fix this muscle fraud: First, be aware that when you see men and women who look unnatural or overly fit in person, on TV, in magazines, and especially on social media, they're more than likely taking steroids and other fitness drugs; it's just that common. And second, if you are a person who takes drugs to attain your fit look, grow some balls and tell the truth, if you can find them that is. We could just drug test everyone, but they would just lie and cheat their way through that as well.

Testing for steroids and other PEDs is nothing but obsolete. The science behind faking and passing steroid tests is as advanced as the drugs themselves. Drug testing in sports and other fitness events is more about appeasement than finding a solution, so the drugs live on. From fake and borrowed urine to diuretics and hard-to-detect HGH, drug users aren't worried one bit about getting caught because most of them are always one step ahead. So how do we catch these cheats? I'm not sure we can catch them or if we even need to. It all goes back to what I said at the very beginning of this book. It's not about people taking drugs, it's about them lying about it at the expense of others who spend their money, hopes, and emotions to achieve what they think is a naturally fit look. It's more about what we can't see that poses most of the problems in fitness, and when you add a little smoke and mirrors to the set, BS takes center stage, and the fraud grows even bigger.

From wonder workouts to miracle machines, the overnight answers to everyone's fitness challenges are just a phone call away, and if you act now, you'll be one of the special people who get an extra bonus of BS. Fitness companies pull out all the stops when they advertise their can't-miss, insta-fit products by using pre-fit models, fake audiences, disappearing ink, and emotional roller coaster testimonials, and it's working. When it comes to any and all fitness advertisements, just remember their number one goal is to make money, not make you healthy. To avoid having to deal with gag-worthy guarantees of another fitness scam, take a closer look at the fine print strategically hidden on the screen; don't fall for the fake tears and miraculous life-changing testimonials; be extra leery of the white-coat endorsements; and remember that Hollywood and its celebrities are built on acting, not health. Speaking of acting, there are a lot of companies and people putting on big shows when it comes to their super supplements and magic pills.

You might not be able to see the big top or the Ferris wheel, or smell the cotton candy, but the carnival is always in town. The strongman, the games of chance on the midway, and the bright lights can always be seen in an advertisement or supplement store near you. Whether it's a supplement salesman, an advertisement on social media, or a graduate from MLM University, they'll all try to pass off their proprietary blends, far-away berries, and super-potent "muscle in a bottle" magic pills as the most amazing things to ever happen in health and wellness. They'll try to sell you with their "studies show" and "scientifically proven" sales pitches, but don't fall for them. When it comes to any and all supplements, transparency is the game. If you are interested in taking a supplement, do your homework: Make a phone call to the manufacturer; ask specific questions about all ingredients in the supplement like amounts and origin; steer clear of proprietary blends (unless they can break it all down for you); and be aware of alternative agendas as with multi-level marketing companies. And above all, steer clear of supplements claiming quick fixes and illness cures. The truth is, if you have a healthy diet, you really shouldn't need supplements. But with the fake and bake ways of our highly unregulated food industry, you have to be really good at spotting food lies, or get ready to be fed a bunch of bull.

Food companies lie, there's just no better way to put it. Oh, they're really good at painting pictures of health on their packages, but much of what is inside those packages is anything but healthy.

You've seen that "All Natural," "Free Range," "Sugar Free," and other labels really don't mean anything, and more than likely, they are hiding dirty truths about how the food was grown or raised. We just can't trust labels, so what do we do? Just like with supplements, we have to know the sources of our foods. We have to either grow our own or actually visit the farms where our foods are grown and get a first-hand look at the entire process. And when we get to those farms, we need to ask a lot of questions. And just like with personal training and supplements, if your questions aren't answered quickly, rationally, and in a specific manner, there's something fishy going on and it's time to leave the farm. Food is a big business—maybe the biggest—and unfortunately, it's made up of a bunch of losers. There's another big business built on the hopes that clients will become big losers, but in a different way, hopefully.

The weight-loss industry is indeed big business, and despite heartfelt testimonials and celebrity feel-good endorsements, they have their scamming skeletons in the closet too.

It's the fad diets that are the worst because they set people up with their overnight disappearing pounds promises, their unhealthy calorie restrictions, and their lack of disclosing that their ten-pounds in two weeks is mostly water. And these types of diets are almost impossible to maintain, so what happens? People stop the diet, go back to eating the way they used to, and the vicious cycle continues. In short, stay away from fad and quick-fix diets; they will leave you worse off than when you started. Although there are sensible diet programs available, there are still questions you should ask about their losing methods. Before you join a weight-loss program, do your research, and find reviews from many different sources about the successes and failures of these programs. Watch out for any program demanding you use their food and their food only, those that add supplements to your diet plan (which they just happen to sell), and any program telling you that exercise is not needed. Regardless of whether or not you join a weight-loss program to lose weight or you plan on going at it alone, do yourself a huge favor: Become nutritionally independent by learning about food—not diets and eating plans—plain old food. Learn about what each type of food does for you, the timing of digestion of different foods, and how your body uses these foods. Once you know these things, you'll know for sure if someone is trying to sell you a big fat lie.

And there you have it. It took me about seventy thousand words to explain to you how fraudulent the healthiest industry in the world really is. Believe me, this book could have easily ended up well over one hundred thousand words, and I will probably end up writing a book on each chapter, but I feel confident that I got my point across. As far as true health, the fitness industry is on its last legs and its last breath, because on the inside, it doesn't resemble anything close to being healthy. From the damaging ways of exercise being taught by our fitness professionals and the overwhelming use and acceptance of drugs, to the fraudulent multi-billion-dollar lies of the supplement and food industry, looks have officially trumped health, and Jack LaLanne is shaking his head at what fitness has become.

Tomorrow I'll get up, eat my breakfast, go train a client, and head to the gym for my workout. I'll walk into the gym, start my warm-up, clear my mind, and get ready to have the best workout I've ever had. And as I go through my workout, I'll watch the healthiest industry in the world do its best to cover up the broken, twisted mess it really is, day after day after day. I'm not sure when the lesson is coming, but if you hear a steroid detector go off in the gym, airport, grocery store, or sporting event, you'll know the real conditioning has begun, and I'll be smiling ear to ear.

Notes

Chapter 1

1. Men's Fitness editors, "The Stupid Things Bad Trainers Say," *Men's Fitness.com*, http://www.mensfitness.com/life/enter-tainment/stupid-things-bad-trainers-say.

Chapter 2

2. Dimity McDowell, "Dangerous Personal Trainers," *Doctors Review.com*, May 2010, http://www.doctorsreview.com/injury-prevention/dangerous-personal-trainers/.

Chapter 3

3. Terry Banawich, "30 Lies of Bodybuilding," *BodyBuilding.com*, January 19, 2017, https://www.bodybuilding.com/fun/30lies.htm.

4. Anthony Roberts, "D-Cups and D-Bol – Women and Anabolic Steroids," *ThinkSteroids.com*, September 9, 2001, https://thinksteroids.com/articles/dbol-women-anabolic-ste-roids/.

5. "What Drugs do Fitness Models Use?" *Nattyornot.com*, October 2, 2014, http://nattyornot.com/drugs-fitness-models-use/.

Chapter 4

6. The Association Against Steroid Abuse, "Trenbolone," *Steroidabuse.com*, http://www.steroidabuse.com/Profiles/trenbolone.html.

7. "Clenbuterol: The Most Popular Hollywood Secret," *NewColonist.com*, http://www.newcolonist.com/clenbuterol/.

8. Todd Zwillich, "Anabolic Steroid Seekers Find Easy Access,"

WebMD, March 18, 2005, http://www.webmd.com/fit-ness-exercise/news/20050318/anabolic-steroid-seek-ers-find-easy-access#1.

Chapter 5

9. The Association Against Steroid Abuse, "Steroid Testing," *Steroidabuse.com,* http://www.steroidabuse.com/steroid-test-ing.html.

10. http://www.testclear.com/Powdered-Urine-Kit-P13.aspx.

Chapter 6

11. Deborah L. Mullen, "How to Spot a Fitness Fraud," *Simplefitnesssolutions.com,* http://www.simplefitnesssolu-tions.com/articles/fitness_frauds.htm.

12. Stephen Propatier, "Joint Pain: Scams, Lies, and Exaggerations, Part 1," *Skeptoid.com,* March 18, 2015, https://skeptoid.com/blog/2015/03/18/joint-pain-part-1/.

Chapter 7

13. Associated Press, "Many Vitamins, Supplements Made by Big Pharmaceutical Companies," *FoxNews.com,* June 10, 2009, http://www.foxnews.com/story/2009/06/10/many-vita-mins-supplements-made-by-big-pharmaceutical-companies. html.

14. "Consumerlab.com Answers," *Consumerlab.com,* January 20, 2015, https://www.consumerlab.com/answers/How+-can+I+find+out+where+a+vitamin+or+supplement+is+-made+and+where+its+ingredients+come+from%2C+-such+as+China+or+the+USA/ where_supplements_come_from/.

15. Robert L. FitzPatrick, "The 10 Big Lies of Multi-Level Marketing," *Falseprofits.com,* https://www.falseprofits.com/ MLM%20Lies.html.

Chapter 8

16. Sydney Lupkin, "5 Gluten Myths You Were Too Embarrassed to Ask About," *ABCNews.go.com,* May 9, 2014, http://abcnews.go.com/Health/gluten-myths-embarrassed/story?id=23645211.

17. https://www.fsis.usda.gov/wps/wcm/connect/fsis-content/internet/main/topics/food-safety-education/get-answers/food-safety-fact-sheets/food-labeling/meat-and-poultry-labeling-terms/meat-and-poultry-labeling-terms.

Chapter 9

18. William Anderson, "4 Top Weight Loss Scams of the Year (So Far)," *Huffingtonpost.com,* January, 29, 2014, (updated) March 31, 2014, http://www.huffingtonpost.com/william-anderson-ma-lmhc/weight-loss-scams_b_4590533.html.

About Bobby Whisnand

Bobby Whisnand is a fitness professional, international keynote speaker, and author who has spent nearly three decades using his knowledge, expertise, and Texas-sized energy to keep the "fit" in fitness.

Endorsed by doctors, surgeons, and other specialists across multiple disciplines — including cardiology, orthopedics, and physical therapy — Whisnand has helped more than 7,000 patients with chronic conditions exercise safely and effectively.

Bobby has multiple certifications as a personal trainer, elite trainer, and specialist in exercise therapy and sports nutrition. Additionally, he has completed two, year-long physical therapy internships and holds a B.S. degree in psychology.

As a keynote speaker, Whisnand has given over 500 presentations on health-related topics and has spoken on behalf of the American Heart Association-Dallas at over 60 events.

His abstract, "Built in America: Making wellness fit for life!" was published in the 2017 *Journal of Obesity and Eating Disorders.*

In addition to creating multiple corporate wellness programs, Bobby has also written numerous other books including *It's All Heart; A Body To Die For: The Painful Truth About Exercise; 12 Rounds: A Day To Day Guide To A Better Life;* and *12 Rounds Exercise Program.*

Take a minute to visit his website for more great information, programs, and products: http://bobbywhisnand.com